YOU 1.0

YOU 1.0

The Ultimate User's Guide for YOU

Includes the 5 P.R.I.M.E. components of
health and wellness

Matthew Kounkel D.C.

iUniverse, Inc.
New York Lincoln Shanghai

YOU 1.0
The Ultimate User's Guide for YOU

iUniverse books may be ordered through booksellers or by contacting:

iUniverse
2021 Pine Lake Road, Suite 100
Lincoln, NE 68512
www.iuniverse.com
1-800-Authors (1-800-288-4677)

ISBN: 0-595-34323-6

Printed in the United States of America

3.5 reasons you should buy this book

1. This book could potentially save you hundreds and thousands of dollars in health care costs.

2. Your health is your most valuable possession, invest in it.

3. This book contains information that you need to operate at your optimal level.

3.5 Your mother wants you too.

Contents

The doctor of the future will give no medicine, but will interest his patients in the care of the human frame, in diet, and in the cause and prevention of disease.
Thomas A. Edison

1.0

YOU 1.0

He who has health has hope; and he who has hope has everything.

Arabian Proverb

Congratulations! Whether you realize it or not, you have just made an investment in yourself. By reading this book, you are arming yourself with knowledge that will help you to lead a more healthy, pain free, and satisfying life. Investing in yourself is the smartest investment you could ever make.

Power on. Clear your hard drive *(brain)* and prepare to save some good information. You are about to read the most important instruction manual ever written.

The instructions for YOU Version 1.0.

YOU 1.0 are the most complex and fascinating object this world has ever seen. YOU 1.0 are more complex than any machine or computer our smartest scientists can dream of. You 1.0 have billions and billions of cells, parts, and pieces, that must all work together in harmony, or else You 1.0 will *crash, become infected with a virus, slow down, become less productive, or simply become outdated.* Humans have been developing and evolving for thousands of years and YOU 1.0 are the product of all of our forbearer's hard work. With proper maintenance You 1.0 can live to be over 100 years old with few, if any problems! Without proper maintenance You 1.0 will become "old and outdated," just like your old Commodore 64 computer system.

You are unique, special, and one of a kind. You are worth "saving" and "backing-up." This owner's manual is going to provide you with the information necessary to keep you running smoothly and trouble free for many years.

Before I go on I want to say one thing. I am not anti-doctor or anti-drug. I wouldn't want to live in a world where I couldn't get the very best healthcare available to myself and my family. If I ever **need** surgery, I want the very best surgeon and pain relief I can afford. If my child ever breaks his/her arm, I want the best orthopedic doctor setting the bone back in place to heal. With that being said, there is something definitely wrong with our system of healthcare. It should not even be called healthcare. That is misleading. It should be called "sick-care" because our healthcare system doesn't "care" for us until we are sick. Unfortunately, most doctors and drugs do very little for our *health*. There is a fundamental lack of prevention and wellness care in our society due to a number of factors including the market, profitability, and our reactive rather than proactive society. We have a backwards medical system. Our medical model waits until we have a "glitch" or a "virus" such as heart disease, cancer, or diabetes and says, "OK, let's see what we can do." We are spending more than ever before on "sick-care" and we seem to be just as sick as ever.

While it is a fact that we are actually healthier than any previous generation, we seem to be overwhelmed with *attention* focused on our health. We live longer, more healthy lives than our grandparents but we hear about health issues in greater numbers and with increasing frequency. News outlets know that health topics sell. You can't watch the 10 o'clock news or pick up a magazine at the grocery store without hearing about the latest epidemic, revolutionary stress reliever, or weight loss program. All of which brings me to the question: If we are living longer, utilizing the latest technological advances, and receiving better medical care than our predecessors, why don't we perceive ourselves as healthier? There is no simple answer to that question. It is my belief that there are a number of contributing factors that have shaped our "health-care" system over the years.

One cause of our negative sense of our healthy selves is that we are a society that likes things NOW! Gone are the slow paced days where you had time for lemonade on the porch with neighbors. We said goodbye to the days when you could go into your doctor's office and shoot the breeze with him/her about your general health concerns many years ago. Gone are the days when you had to go home to call someone, and at the same time they had to be home to answer the phone! With all of the technological advances we have witnessed in the last 20 years we have become accustomed to immediate results. If you want to talk to someone, call their cell phone. We don't even bother to try them at home any more. Let's face it, who spends any time at home? If you can't get their cell phone, try their email. No luck? Try their pager. Not fast enough? Use your Blackberry. No dice? Two-way them. And so on and so on.

We have become a society where convenience equals quickness. If you don't have 30 seconds to spare to run into the gas station to pay for gas, simply pay at the pump. Can't wait two days for an important document to be delivered by the post office? Fax it. No time to research your term paper at the library? Find your information on the web. Easier still, find a term paper on the web, copy and paste it, write your name at the top, and you are done. All of this technology is wonderful and I doubt anyone of us would sincerely wish to live without it. I have a cell phone, I pay at the pump, I did not copy and paste this book however. Where we run into problems is when we wish to apply this hurry up style to better ourselves. It has taken years for you to become you. No matter how fast information travels over phone lines or up to bounce off of satellites, our bodies and minds cannot enjoy the benefits of immediate transformation. We cannot copy and paste our health. On the one hand that would be terrific. I could walk into a gym, work out for an hour or so, and walk out looking like Arnold Schwarzenegger in his prime. But, on the other hand, I am pretty happy that my fat cells don't immediately expand after every piece of pie I eat.

Immediacy has had a negative impact on our healthcare system as well. Healthcare providers are sometimes forced by the public to treat the effects of a problem rather than the cause. We take chemicals developed and designed by pharmaceutical companies to lower our high blood pressure. Forget about exercising or modifying your eating habits; that would take to much time and effort. If you get headaches from slouching in front of a computer terminal all day; forget about stretching or modifying your workstation to suit your particular size. Simply deal with it and take a couple of pills. It is this mentality that is reducing healthcare to an application of chemistry. It is not a lack of Advil™ in your system that is causing headaches, or that your body doesn't produce enough Lipitor™ and that is why your cholesterol level is too high. (*Again let me reiterate that drugs and medicine when used properly and ethically are wonderful things.*) We have become a society that wants our health and we want it with as little effort as possible, and we want it NOW!

This desire for a "magic pill" shows. According to a recent study, Americans averaged about 11 prescriptions per capita in 2003.[1] That is almost 3 billion prescriptions filled in 1 year in the U.S. alone! We have become a society of quick fix and chemical junkies.

Why do we feel that chemistry is the answer to all of our health concerns? In part, it is due to the wonderful life saving advances medicine has made in the last 100 years. Vaccines have saved countless lives. Insulin can provide a diabetic with a near normal lifestyle. Even aspirin can provide temporary relief to arthritis sufferers. Because of these amazing advances we have come to the belief that chemistry must be the answer to all of our prayers.

This dependence upon chemistry for our health can be costly however, and not just in dollar signs. Millions of people every year have adverse drug reactions. Almost 2 million people per year have drug complications that result in 180,000 deaths or life threatening illness according to one major study. People are dying or getting sick from taking too many pills, in too high a dosage, for too long, for conditions where they will see little to no benefit from taking the drug.

Unfortunately, our society and a majority of our current health care system (think "sick care") ignore the simple, effective, and low cost treatment options outlined in this book. Our "sick care" insurance system is set up to reimburse you for drugs and visits to the doctors office after you are already sick, not a gym membership or counseling with a nutritionist. Our "sick care" health system's focus is directed towards new, expensive drugs and surgeries to combat pain, insomnia, obesity and a host of other ailments that are largely preventable in the first place.

Studies have shown that simple lifestyle changes can have a dramatic impact on your health. Choices such as smoking, a poor diet, drinking too much alcohol, and lack of exercise are responsible for 80% of one's risk of heart disease and almost 100% of the risk for developing diabetes. Instead of hearing about living a healthy lifestyle however, we are inundated with commercials and ads promoting the next "miracle" drug. The medical establishment is set up to be reactive to problems, and not proactive to stop them from becoming problems in the first place, and the pharmaceutical companies, with their $25 billion a year marketing budgets, are banking on it. This issue will not likely go away soon. The medical establishment, insurance companies, and even lawyers have a huge stake in what happens to the health of our country. If we were more responsible for our own health, took proper preventative measures, and didn't expect the "quick fix" for our problems, our entire healthcare system would be forced to change.

The purpose of this book is not to scare you away from doctors and drugs. The purpose of this book is to show you that true health comes from the "inside-out," not the "outside-in." Prevention is the key to establishing and maintaining health and wellness. We need to install our own "anti-virus" protection BEFORE we get sick. You must have a solid "operating system" if you want to live a healthy, problem free life. Luckily, being healthy isn't nearly as complicated as your computer's operating system. You just need to ask yourself, "What kind of operating system am I currently running on?" Are you running on a high stress, low exercise, poor nutrition operating system? If so, you are setting yourself up for system failure. If, however, you have a solid operating system based on the PRIME components of wellness you are more likely to assure yourself of a problem and "glitch free" life.

> ### The PRIME operating system for YOU 1.0
> The PRIME operating system for YOU 1.0 is a fully integrated system consisting of the following components: Posture, Rest, Intake, Mind, and Exercise, the 5 cornerstones to health and wellness. Within this user's guide you will learn why each of these components is critical to your well-being and how to optimize each of these components for YOU 1.0.

We are lucky enough to live during a wondrous time in history. We have witnessed things that our ancestors never dreamed possible. Technology is changing everything in our lives at an incredible pace. It makes things faster, better, more convenient, and easier. The problem with technology is that the human body was not designed to adapt as quickly. Your body takes time to heal and grow. Some day we may be able to zap our cells and bodies to change more quickly, to stimulate growth, healing, and pain reduction. Someday, we may be able to insert a chip under our skin and download the latest anti-bacterial and anti-virus software into us! Until that day comes, it is ultimately up to each one of us to respond appropriately and responsibly to better our health and well-being.

This book is an instruction manual for YOU 1.0. In this book you will learn about the 5 components that make up the PRIME operating system of wellness for YOU 1.0.

Posture

Rest

Intake

Mind

Exercise

What makes this book different from other books is that we will examine not only HOW your body works, but WHY it works the way it does. Some examples of what is to come include: How and why we gain weight, what we can do to minimize weight gain, and even how to lose weight. (Hint-dieting alone just won't work.) What happens when we exercise and why it is good for us. Why do we need rest and sleep and what are the best ways to get it. What does stress do to your body and what can we do about it, and much more. Once we understand the HOW and the WHY of YOU 1.0 we can take steps to achieve maximum efficiency and make YOU 1.0 the best it can be.

References

1. Kaiser Family Foundation, August 30, 2004.

2.0

POSTURE

To live a long, energetic, active life, few things matter more than good posture.
The Rejuvenation Factor by Calliet and Gross

What does posture have to do with anything?

That is a good question. But first let's look at what posture is. Posture is defined as the position of our body or body parts. Therefore, by definition we can have good or bad posture depending on what is defined as normal. More on that in a moment.

For thousands of years posture has been used as a measuring stick of health and vitality, but in this day and age it is more often associated with the arts rather than the sciences. Posture is often associated with beauty and grace from runway models to statues and paintings of the human form. On a subconscious level we also use posture as a barometer of health. When you stand up straight you seem healthier even if you are not. A stooped over and slouched posture is not something we think about when we picture a healthy, vital human being. If I asked you to picture a healthy person right now, someone you work with or a friend or relative; what do they look like in your mind's eye? Are they stooped over and bent? Are they sitting or lying down when you picture them? Probably not. Most people, whether they know it or not, picture a healthy person as someone who is standing upright, with their shoulders back, seemingly impervious to the constant downward pull of gravity. It seems rather ironic then, that this mirror image of our health for thousands of years, our posture, is virtually ignored by modern day physicians. Too often we want to delve into the minute and sub-molecular levels of our bodies to determine the causes of our problems. We ignore the global or whole body problems that are right in front of our noses.

At this point you may be saying, "Yeah, yeah, posture may be important, that's why my mother always told me to sit up straight, but it is not as important as my diet, or exercise, or rest right?" Read on.

<u>Just how important is our posture?</u>

Posture is *just* as important as eating right, exercising, getting a good nights sleep, and avoiding potentially harmful substances like alcohol, drugs, and tobacco. Good posture is a way of doing things with more energy, less stress and fatigue. The importance of good posture in an overall fitness program is often overlooked by fitness advisors and fitness seekers alike. In fact, the benefits of good posture may be among the best kept secrets of the current health movement. The good news is that almost everyone can avoid the problems caused by bad posture, and YOU 1.0 can make improvements at any age.

Good posture means that your bones are properly aligned and your muscles, joints, and ligaments can work as nature intended. It means that your vital organs are in the right position and can function at peak efficiency. Good posture also helps contribute to the normal functioning of your nervous system. Oh yeah! You know that pain and stiffness between your shoulder blades and up into your neck? Good posture can help that as well.

To understand why posture is so important we must dig a little into physics. For those of you who just dropped the book to the ground shuddering at the thought of your high school physics class, please continue. I promise it won't be painful. Especially if you sit up straight!

On earth, and everywhere in the universe for that matter, there is a force called gravity. That's right, the thing Sir Isaac Newton discovered when an apple fell from a tree and hit him on the head. Gravity, it seems, is a constant and relentless force that is constantly pulling down on us towards the center of the earth. It doesn't change much for us surface dwellers, and whether you like it or not it affects virtually every living thing on the planet, including you. Gravity affects the way we stand, sit, walk, run, and even how we sleep. It can be blamed for the majority of back problems and postural problems that we see everyday: Herniated discs from twisting and lifting heavy objects, forward head posture (more on that in a minute), and muscle strains and sprains from overexertion. But let's not play the blame game with poor old gravity, it can't help itself, that is what it does throughout the universe.

In order to understand how gravity affects us we need to get back to physics for a moment. Let's try a little experiment. Grab something that weighs about 10 pounds, (about the weight of your head incidentally.) It can be virtually anything you can hold in one hand: A full milk jug, a dumbbell, or my favorite, a bowling ball. Now, hold this object in one hand and place your elbow on something solid like a table or counter. Make sure your forearm is straight up and down and hold this object for 3 minutes. Are you done already? Did your arm tire out? Probably not, but your elbow may be sore. OK, this time you can put some padding under your elbow and let's try this again. Only this time bend your arm so the object and your arm are at about a 45 degree angle. Now hold for 3 minutes. Could you do it? Was it a little harder this time? Of course it was.

What you created was what your physics professor called a lever arm. When your arm was straight up and down the entire force of the object and gravity was transmitted through your entire arm down to the elbow. When the angle was introduced, you now had to use muscles, tendons, and ligaments to hold up the object and your forearm. In other words, you are very similar to a building made of bricks. When the bricks are stacked directly on top of each other the structure is very strong and stable. If the bricks are offset just a little bit you get cracking and an unstable building.

WHICH ARE YOU?
THE EMPIRE STATE BUILDING OR THE LEANING
TOWER OF PISA?

Let's transfer this new found physics knowledge to your wonderfully magnificent body. As we are developing inside our mother's womb one of the very first things that researchers can identify is our spinal column and spinal cord. These things begin to form before any other organs or tissues are formed; which makes them pretty important in my book. As the embryo continues to develop we start to see our vertebral column take a C shaped form. By the time we are born we have a lumbar curve (low back) and thoracic curve (mid-back), while our cervical curve (neck) takes a few months after birth to develop. We are born perfect by design. By the time we are walking, roughly age one, we have developed our familiar "S" shaped curve that we know and love. Now what is the importance of these curves? Well, our spinal curves serve us by acting as shock absorbers. Every time we move, we are placing physical stress on our joints including the joints in our back and spine. If our spine was a straight line it wouldn't be able to absorb shock as well as a curved structure and still maintain its shape.

The S shape of our spine also gives us some much needed slack for our very important spinal cord. Your spinal cord is a bundle of nerves that lives in the middle of your vertebral column and sends individual nerves to all the different parts of your body and back again to your brain. Without our S shaped spine we wouldn't have the slack we need to bend over at the waist to pick up "Junior" or to crane our necks upward to look at the stars.

So, we've got this spring-like S shaped curved vertebral column that is supported by all of our muscles and ligaments which act like guy wires and struts that keep us from falling over. Do you think that more stress is put on these guy wires if you lean over or if you have bad posture? Of course. Now just to be clear, these guy wires and struts are living tissues, muscles, ligaments, and tendons. All of which are pain sensitive and susceptible to fatigue and wear and tear. I know what you're thinking. You're thinking that "I've read 12 ½ pages of this book so far, and all I have been told is that bad posture can cause some pain and muscle tightness?" But wait, there's more. Much more.

According to the *American Journal of Pain Management* "Posture affects and moderates every physiological function from breathing to hormone production. Spinal pain, headaches, mood, blood pressure, pulse, and lung capacity are among the functions most easily influenced by posture. Ultimately, it appears that homeostasis, and autonomic regulations are intimately connected with posture."[1] Wow! Please read that again.

"Posture affects and moderates every physiological function."

That is quite a bold statement from a respected medical journal. So why is it that your mother and I are the only ones that are preaching the benefits of maintaining good posture? Good question. Hopefully, after you read this chapter you will help to spread the word as well. Let's get back to that statement above from the *American Journal of Pain Management.* Whenever I tell someone that posture affects more than just back muscles, they invariably have a hard time believing it. Posture can affect your lung capacity? Your hormone production? Your mood? Yes, yes, and yes. Unfortunately it is rather difficult to measure your hormone levels or your mood through a book, so I will try to do the next best thing. I want you to do these next four exercises-and don't cheat. I think you will be amazed. These "Show and Feel" tests were first demonstrated to me in April of 1999 by Dr. Mark Charette D.C. of Las Vegas, Nevada. He has been examining posture and the feet for many years and is one of the best extremity chiropractors in the world.

The most common abnormal posture in our society is forward head translation, which is also called anterior head translation, or positive Z-axis translation of the head. This is seen when your head is in front of shoulders. Because this is a very easy posture to duplicate, and it is the most common posture abnormality, we will use anterior head translation for our tests.

Please stand up and pretend that your chin is resting on train tracks and can only move in two directions, front and back. Now, jut your head straight forward as far in front of your shoulders as you can. Next, take in a deep a breath and notice how much air you can bring in. Bring your head back to its neutral position directly over your shoulders. Take in as deep a breath as you can. Did you notice a difference? You may have noticed that you could take a deeper breath and hold more air when your head was in the posturally correct position.

Let's try another one. Jut your head out in front of your shoulders just like before, only this time instead of taking in a deep breath, turn your head from side to side like you are checking for traffic at a stop sign. Now, bring your head back over your shoulders and turn your head from side to side. Did you notice a difference this time?

How about another? I know you are having fun, and even if you're not, if anyone else is in the room they are certainly enjoying themselves by watching you. Okay, same drill as before, head out in front of you. This time look up toward the ceiling until your head stops. Bring your head back over your shoulders and repeat looking at the ceiling. Could you look up easier and farther the second time?

Okay, one final "Show and Feel" test. Like before, jut your head out in front of your body. This time, with your arms starting at your sides, raise them up and away from you like you were going to touch the backs of your hands together above your head. Notice where your arms naturally stop. Now bring your head back over your shoulders and repeat. Your arms don't stop at the same place do they? You probably had a greater range of motion during the second part of the test than during the first part of the test didn't you? What did we accomplish during the last 3 minutes, besides making you look like a goofball? Well, hopefully you started to realize that your posture may be more important than you may have realized, AND that you should have listened to your mother more often.

These four simple "Show and Feel" tests demonstrate how a seemingly innocent thing like posture can affect your lung capacity and your range of motion, not to mention how much harder your muscles must work to hold your head up. It has been estimated that for every inch forward your ear is from the middle of your shoulder you lose approximately 18-20% of your lung capacity. No wonder you are tired! Not only are your muscles working overtime to support your head but they may not be receiving the oxygen they need to function efficiently.

As we noted earlier, poor posture affects much more than we may know. We have already shown that posture can affect our lung capacity and our range of motion. Poor posture also causes fatigue. Earlier we talked about physics and lever arms. Well it shouldn't be too difficult to imagine that the more abnormal our posture is the more our muscles have to work to keep us upright. The harder our muscles work the more energy they use, which in turn wears them out faster. Not only can we become more easily fatigued but poor posture can cause tight, achy muscles in the neck, back, arms, and legs. In fact more than 80% of neck and back problems are the result of tight, achy muscles brought on by years of bad posture.

Poor posture can also cause joint stiffness and pain. Recent research in the journal *Spine* has indicated that the natural curves of your spine are adversely affected by fatigue associated with poor posture.[2] The result of these abnormal spinal curves can cause uneven stresses on joints leading to degenerative arthritis which leads to pain. Poor posture, improper spinal biomechanics, and limited joint mobility increase the likelihood of arthritis and associated conditions as we age.

Effects of Poor Posture

- Poor posture can cause headaches and jaw pain.
- Postural fatigue of the neck not only causes tight and achy muscles, but it also affects your balance. Much like in people who suffer from chronic neck pain or whiplash.[3]
- Poor posture can cause obstructive sleep apnea and difficulty sleeping.

- Posture has been linked to arm pain and overuse injuries such as muscle strains and ligament sprains.
- Some researchers "postulate" that poor posture can cause heart and lung disorders, digestive problems, upper abdominal pain, and chronic fatigue because of the compression of certain organs and body parts due to a stooped posture.
- Poor posture has been linked to impaired creative thinking and emotional control, and has been shown to decrease your reaction time in certain instances.[4]
- Poor posture can also lead to low back pain which is one of the most prevalent and difficult problems to treat in this country. Low back pain is so common that it is the number 2 cause of lost workdays in the United States, just behind the common cold!
- Some research has shown that poor posture may decrease endorphin production, your body's own natural pain fighting hormones.

Now that we have talked about some of the dangers of poor posture, it is time to examine what good posture looks like. Because bad posture can take almost any form, we have a standard or "normal" that we can measure against it. Incidentally, the most common form of bad posture that I see every day is the forward head, shoulders rounded forward, and arched or rounded lower back. (Remember, just because it's common does not mean it's normal.) Normal posture from the front is considered to be: eyes or tops of ears level, shoulders level, hips level, and knee caps level. You should also be able to draw a straight line from a spot between your eyes to your breast bone, to your pubic bone, down to a spot in-between both of your feet. From the side, perfect posture looks like this: Your "external auditory meatus" (Let's use ear hole from now on, Okay?) should be directly above the boney bump on top of your shoulder, also known as your AC joint. Your AC joint should be above your hip or the head of your big leg bone called the femur which should be above the middle of the side of your knee. This line should continue down to end just in front of the boney bump on the outside of your ankle. That is perfect posture. To see how you "stack-up," look into a mirror for your front view or have a friend examine you from the front and the side.

How Did This Happen?

If we are born perfect by design, how does poor posture happen? It can happen from accidents, slips and falls, or almost any tissue damaging trauma that permanently alters your body in someway. However, poor posture most commonly develops due to environmental factors or bad habits. The good news is that you have a lot of control. The bad news is that our bodies don't seem to be adapting as fast as technology is advancing, and in some cases this may be a problem. Today, posture related problems are increasing due to the following factors:

✓ We are a society that sits and watches more television than any previous generation. Some reports suggest that we watch at least 5 hours a day.
✓ We are becoming a more electronic society, with more and more people working at sedentary desk jobs or sitting in front of computer terminals.
✓ More and more cars are crowding our roads, resulting in accidents and injuries and also resulting in longer drive times in cars with poorly designed seats.

In most cases, poor posture results from a combination of several factors, which can include the following:

1. Careless sitting, standing, sleeping habits.

2. Poor sleep support.—We spend almost ½ of our lives sleeping, often on a mattress that is poorly suited to our body type.

3. Excessive weight.—Where we carry our extra pounds can affect how we carry ourselves and our posture.

4. Visual difficulties.—We squint and crane our necks at the computer because we haven't had time to get our eyes checked.

5. Emotional difficulties.—Depression, anxiety, and stress, as well as other psychological problems can have a tremendous impact on our posture. Unfortunately, they also contribute to a negatively reinforcing cycle which is hard to break out of. When we are depressed we may feel like we have the weight of the world on our shoulders, bowing our heads to stress and rounding our shoulders forward. This posture also reflects the negative image of self worth which subconsciously reinforces the feelings of depression or stress.

6. Foot problems or improper shoes.—High heeled shoes for women play havoc on the lower back.

7. Weak muscles or muscle imbalance.—Some neurological problems or muscle problems which only affect certain areas or a specific side (say a stroke for example), can have a negative impact on the way we are able to carry ourselves, which can result in muscle wasting and joint deterioration.

8. Accidents, injuries and falls.—As mentioned before, tissue damage from a slip, trip, fall, or any type of accident can permanently alter our biomechanics if not treated properly, and can result in permanent postural impairments.

9. Negative self image, especially in female teenagers.—This topic could be included in the emotional difficultly section, but I wanted to pay special attention to it here. It is unfortunate in our society that appearances are so important to social stature, but no-where is this more apparent than in teenage females. They are at an awkward stage in life, where they are growing faster than their male counterparts, and in some cases even faster than their close friends. Because of this they may subconsciously slouch or exaggerate their forward head posture to disguise the fact that they are growing taller. They may also be maturing sexually at a quicker pace than their friends (and almost certainly faster than the boys their age) and are developing breasts. We can be a cruel species and pick on others that are different from ourselves. Therefore, some young females may roll their shoulders forward, again not consciously, in an effort to hide the fact that they are maturing into women. Once these postural habits are formed and reinforced over a period of weeks, months, or even years, they are very difficult to reverse and correct.

10. Occupational stress and a poorly designed work environment.—Ergonomics is a buzzword for today and it couldn't have happened too soon. Office workers who must crook a phone to their ear while they jot down notes or who sit at a desk or workstation that was set up for someone twice their size may very well pay for these poorly designed work environments with their health.

10.5. Anatomic abnormalities.—Scoliosis, one leg shorter than another, and other diseases and genetic abnormalities are rare but they can contribute greatly to how one's posture will develop.

OK, we discussed 10.5 common causes of poor posture and we covered some of the consequences that poor posture has on YOU 1.0. Now let's take a look at how we can improve our posture and ultimately ourselves.

References

1. Lennon, J. Shealy, CN, Cady, RK, Mattia, W, Cox, R, Simpson, WF *American Journal of Pain Management*. Vol 4 Na 1, Jan 1994.

2. Orloff, Heidi A. PhD; Rapp, Catherine M. BS *The Effects of Load Carriage on Spinal Curvature and Posture*. Spine. 29(12):1325-1329, June 15, 2004.

3. Guy Gosselin, Hamid Rassoulianb and Ian Browna. *Effects of neck extensor muscles fatigue and balance*. Clinical Biomechanics. Volume 19, Issue 5, June 2004, Pages 473-479.

4. Cooper, Robert, *High Energy Living*. Rosedale Press, 2000.

3.0

Improving Posture

All parts of the body which have a function if used in moderation and exercised in labors in which each is accustomed, become thereby healthy, well developed, and age more slowly, but if unused they become liable to disease, defective in growth, and age quickly.

Hippocrates

The first step to improve your posture is to determine where you may have problems. Stand relaxed in front of a mirror with your feet about shoulder width apart. Make sure that you are standing square to the mirror. Take a few steps in place, close your eyes, and nod your head up and down a few times. Open your eyes and check your posture. Check to make sure your eyes are level as well as your shoulders. Observe if your head is slightly rotated or if your shoulders are slightly rotated. If your head is rotated one ear may be more visible in the mirror than the other. See if your arms are the same distance away from your body and if your hands reach the same point on your hips. Is one hand higher than the other? If so, your shoulders may not be level.

> Quick Posture Self Check
> Stand with your heels about 3 inches apart and your back, rear, and head touching the wall. Put your hand behind your neck and your low back. You should be able to move your hand but there should not be more than 1 inch from the wall to your neck or low back.

To check your side profile you will need the help of a friend. Stand relaxed again, take a few steps, nod your head up and down and stop in a relaxed position. Have your friend look at your ear hole and see if it is directly above your shoulder joint. Your shoulder joint should be directly above your hip joint which should be above the middle of your knee. Next, the middle of your knee should be slightly in front of the boney bump on your ankle. An easy way to check your side profile is to use a piece of colored string hanging from the ceiling. With someone helping you, all of the points described above should fall along this line.

In addition to evaluating your standing posture, notice the way that you sit at a desk or at your computer. You may need to make some adjustments to your workstation to promote the posture you need.

Some postural deviations may be very slight and hard to notice. Have a chiropractor or physical therapist observe you if you have any questions. They will probably recommend some stretches and exercises you can perform to improve your posture as well.

INSTANT POSTURE DOWNLOADS...

At your workplace:

♦   Evaluate your workplace. If you sit at a computer for most of the day check your workstation for ergonomic correctness.

If you sit at work:

- Use a chair with firm low back support. Sit up with your back straight and your shoulders back. Your buttocks should touch the back of your chair. Use a rolled up towel or back support to maintain the proper curves in your back.
- Adjust your chair so that your desk or table is elbow high. Your forearms should be parallel with the floor while typing.
- Use a foot rest to keep pressure off of your lower back and legs. With your feet flat on the floor, you should be able to slide four fingers in between the underside of your thigh and the chair.
- Take "Micro-breaks." Get up and stretch frequently, every half-hour or so if you sit for long periods of time. You don't need to spend 10-15 minutes stretching, just 30 seconds or so to loosen up the muscles that have been resting idle for so long. Raise your arms above your head, try to touch your shoulder blades together, and reach down and touch your toes. This will keep your muscles from tightening up throughout the day.
- Keep your computer screen about 15 degrees below eye level. This position allows you to sit comfortably with your eyes in a position that causes the least amount of fatigue.
- Place reference or typing material on a stand close to and even with the computer screen.
- Have your eyes examined. Poor eyesight can cause eye fatigue and force you to unconsciously squint and crane your neck in order to see the screen in front of you.

If you stand at work:

- Wear comfortable shoes with good arch support.
- Give your low back a break by putting one foot up on a box or step and alternating between the two legs.
- Hold your head high, chin firmly forward, shoulders back, chest out, and stomach tucked in to increase your balance.
- Take breaks and sit every 3-4 hours.
- When lifting, let your legs do the work. Stand close to the object and where possible, squat down and straddle it. Grasp the object and slowly lift the load by straightening your legs as you stand up. Carry the object close to your body. (Remember your center of gravity?) Set the object down in the same way. We all seem to know how to pick an object up, but after carrying it a

while we get tired and we forget how to set it down. Many low back injuries occur during this phase.

◆   When bending, never twist from the waist and bend forward at the same time. In other words, stand squarely in front of the object you are picking up. Bend your knees and keep your back straight.

In the car:

◆   Adjust your seat so that your knees are slightly higher than your hips.
◆   Adjust your seat forward or back so that when your hands are in the 10 and 2 o'clock position (remember back to driver's Ed?) your forearms and upper arms create a 90 degree angle.
◆   Remove your wallet, if you carry one, so that you are not sitting on top of it. This will help to keep your pelvis level.
◆   Move the rear-view mirror so that it faces the ceiling. Now, adjust your seat so that you are leaning back at about a 15 degree angle. Make sure that your low back is supported as you sit up straight, and your head should rest on the head rest. Next, re-adjust your rearview mirror so that you can see out of the rear window. This is the position you should find yourself in most of the time. Every time you look in the rearview mirror you should be able to see clearly out of the back. This will help to remind you to sit in this position.

While sleeping:

◆   Make sure that your head is level with the rest of your spine. When on your back, your neck should be supported as well as your head. When on your side, your head should be level with the rest of your spine.
◆   Avoid too many or very thick pillows. This is the equivalent of watching TV on the couch with your head propped against the armrest for 6-8 hours. Use a thin pillow with a small pillow under your neck instead, or buy a pillow customized for you.
◆   Don't sleep on your stomach. Stomach sleeping forces your head into rotation for extended periods of time. Imaging turning your head to the left and keeping it there for 4 or more hours! You can see how you might wake up with a stiff neck if you are a stomach sleeper.

More Tips to Optimize Your Posture

Keep your weight down

As we talked about earlier, adding weight to your frame shifts your center of gravity which makes your muscles and joints work harder. This speeds up the rate of degeneration and makes you tire more easily. Ways to keep your weight down will be discussed more thoroughly in the following chapters.

Exercise

Start a regular exercise program that incorporates posture improving techniques as well as a cardiovascular workout. Regular exercise keeps you flexible and

> **Yoga and Pilates**
> Yoga, Pilates, or any other "core" strengthening exercise regime, is a great way to build strength and endurance within your posture muscles. These types of exercise also help to stretch tissues that become chronically shortened as we age. This strengthening and stretching of specific muscles helps to create a balance within your muscle groups.

helps tone your muscles to support proper posture. Stretch and strengthen your core muscles which help to maintain your upright posture during the day. Typical core exercises include: abdominal exercises (crunches, sit-ups, etc.), back arching, giant ball exercises, and many more.

Get a massage

Massages are a great way to become more in touch with your body. Massage directly influences your nervous and muscular systems, enabling you to release chemicals that may have built up in your body in response to the stressors and postural imbalances encountered in life. When these chemicals linger in the body for prolonged periods we feel stiff and achy, we can get seriously ill, or we can become susceptible to pain and injury.

When you have a postural dysfunction your tissues must work harder to keep you upright. These tissues become more easily fatigued and wear out more quickly than normal. They also produce chemicals that your body has a hard time expelling. Massage can help your body to get rid of these toxins and restore a proper balance to your structural tissues.

Go to your chiropractor

Your doctor of chiropractic is trained to diagnose and treat musculoskeletal conditions including conditions related to posture. For more information on chiropractic see below.

What is Chiropractic?

Chiropractic, as a profession, has been around since the late 1800's but records show that the practice of chiropractic has been around much longer. The first recorded adjustment of the spine was found in ancient kung fu writings dating back to 2650 B.C. In 1500 B.C. the first low back adjustment was recorded in Greece, and in 500 B.C. Hippocrates, "the Father of Modern Medicine," wrote two works on spinal adjusting and the nervous system.

The word "Chiropractic" comes from the Greek word Chiropraktikos, meaning "effective treatment by hand." Chiropractic is based on the following principles: 1. The body is a self-regulatory and self-healing organism. 2. The nervous system is the master system that regulates and controls all other organs and tissues of the body and relates the individual to his/her environment. 3. Spinal biomechanical dysfunction in the form of vertebral subluxation complex may affect the nervous system's ability to regulate function. In other words, if a spinal segment is out of alignment or is not moving correctly, it can negatively affect your nervous system. 4. It is the focus of the doctor of chiropractic to correct, manage, or minimize vertebral subluxation through a spinal adjustment.[1] In other words, most chiropractors believe that if the nervous system is operating correctly your body is able to heal and repair itself. We are all born with an inborn ability to heal ourselves, a so called "internal physician," which is controlled by our nervous system. If there is some type of interference affecting the nervous system you are more susceptible to health problems, pain, and potential disease. One area that can influence nervous system function is your spine. The boney structure or vertebral column that protects your spinal cord is the primary area where your nerves can be affected.

Current chiropractic research focuses more on the nervous system than the bones that protect it. Scientists have only recently begun to understand how our bodies react to musculoskeletal pain and how the chiropractic adjustment helps to alleviate that pain. One theory is that the chiropractic adjustment stimulates specific nerves which sense the position and motion of a joint. If these nerves are activated with a specific stimulus that is high enough but not so high that there is tissue damage, the nerves signaling pain will decrease their rate of fire, in essence decreasing the amount of pain you feel. You have probably done this yourself but may not have realized it at the time. If you have ever stubbed your toe and hopped up and down on one foot you have activated a similar response. This instinctive maneuver activates millions of motion and position neurons which help to lower the sensation of pain in the stubbed toe.

Chiropractic is mainly thought of as a treatment method for musculoskeletal complaints and pain. Back pain, neck pain, extremity disorders and pain, and headaches usually respond extremely well with careful chiropractic treatment. Other non-musculoskeletal disorders, such as colic and asthma, have reportedly been treated successfully with chiropractic treatment but further research is needed to validate these claims.

Chiropractors act as assistants to your internal physician and attempt to reduce interference to your nervous system so that it can operate correctly. Chiropractic is the science of finding areas of your nervous system that aren't working properly, the art of correcting or reducing the impact these dysfunctional areas have on your nervous system, and the philosophy that you have an extraordinary ability to heal yourself when allowed to naturally.

References

1. *The Chiropractic Paradigm, the Cleveland Perspective*. Cleveland Chiropractic College.

4.0

REST

No day is so bad it can't be fixed with a nap.

Carrie Snow

The second component to the PRIME operating system for wellness is Rest. Within the PRIME operating system rest can take many forms, including sleep and relaxation. In our hectic lifestyles rest is often neglected. We sacrifice our rest for other more "important" things. We rush around trying to get all of our tasks accomplished, only to come home at the end of a long day and fall onto the couch in front of the TV to *rest*. The next day we get up after 5-6 hours of sleep and do it all over again, and again and again. The human body is like any other operating system, it can't go at full power for 24 hours a day, 7 days a week, 365 days a year even if you want it to. Rest is crucial to your survival and well-being. Let's take a look at rest and what it means to you.

Sleep

One of the most important aspects of rest is sleep. Sleep is defined as unconsciousness from which the person can be aroused by sensory or other stimuli.[1] In other words, you are unconscious to the world around you, but yet, you can be easily woken by stimulating one of your 5 senses if the stimulus is strong enough. Most of us need 7-9 hours of sleep per night to operate at our best. When we don't receive the rest and sleep we need we may become cranky, lethargic, and unable to focus clearly. Why this happens is not clearly understood. While we all know that we need to rest and sleep, researchers are not exactly sure why.

Sleep causes two major types of physiological effects: The first physiological effect of sleep acts upon your nervous system and the second on the other structures of the body. Sleep seems to be most important to your master system or your nervous system. Research has shown that a person with a severed spinal cord in the neck shows no harmful effects in the body beneath the level of nerve damage that can be attributed to a sleep and wakefulness cycle.[2] This means that the lack of a sleep-wake cycle does not seem to harm your organs and body systems, except for your brain. This does NOT mean that the remainder of your body doesn't need rest, only that it doesn't necessarily need *sleep*. We have all experienced a reduced mental capacity at the end of a busy day. We are unable to concentrate, our mind wanders, and we become irritable if we don't get the rest our brain needs. Researchers aren't sure why this happens but the most widely accepted theory is that our brains need to re-establish a baseline between the different parts of the nervous system.

We are constantly processing information and interpreting stimuli every second we are awake (even to a lessor degree while we sleep!) It is thought that when we sleep we are able to purge some of the useless data that we accumulate throughout the day. During the typical day we are constantly being bombarded with stimuli, most of which we don't even realize. Colors, sights, background noise, smells, tastes, positions, and textures to name a few. The shirt you are wearing now is resting on millions of pressure and touch receptors which you were probably unaware of, unless your shirt is itchy and irritating! It is thought that sleep lets our brain "turn-off" most of these sensory areas in order to file away the more important memories of the day. Sleep acts like *control-alt-delete* for our brains, resetting us to prepare for the onslaught of sensory input we will experience the next day. After resetting your system and waking up, you can start the next day without all of the junk clogging up your hard drive and slowing you down.

Sleep also allows our brain to replenish important neurotransmitters that are used up during the day processing all of the stimuli we are exposed to. These neurotransmitters are essential for learning and memory. Preventing the supply from building back up because of poor sleep or lack of sleep interferes with the ability to learn and remember.[3]

The second physiological effect of sleep influences the other structures of the body. When we sleep our sympathetic nervous system becomes less active and our parasympathetic nervous system activity increases. What this means is that our digestive activity may increase, our skeletal muscle tone is decreased and enters a mainly relaxed state, our blood pressure falls slightly, and our metabolic rate drops by 10-30 per cent. Blood flow increases to the deeper muscles in our bodies and our metabolism slows, this allows repair to take place to our cells and organs.

Our immune system seems to be directly linked to sleep as well. A lack of sleep decreases our ability to fend off bacteria and viral attacks. Studies have linked a decrease in natural killer cells found throughout our tissues when we don't get enough sleep. Natural killer cells are white blood cells that hunt down and destroy invading bacteria and viruses. We also know that our immune system can control how sleepy we feel. Cytokines, which are present in the blood system and moderate inflammatory conditions, make you sleepy. We have all had a cold or the flu when we just couldn't get out of bed. These cytokines and other factors cause the feeling of tiredness, which allows your immune system to operate at peak efficiency to destroy the invaders. Whatever the reason we need sleep, we know that we cannot do without it.

Sleep is usually categorized into two different types: Slow wave sleep and REM sleep. We cycle between the two different types of sleep throughout the night. Slow wave sleep, which is called this because our brain waves and activity is very slow, is often thought of as "dream-less" sleep. This is not actually the case, it has been shown that dreams do occur during this phase but they are rarely remembered. Slow wave sleep is typically very restful and during slow wave sleep our blood pressure, metabolic rate, and respiration rate drops.

REM sleep, or Rapid Eye Movement sleep, occurs between periods of slow wave sleep, about every 90 minutes, and lasts between 5-30 minutes. When you are very tired your REM sleep is quite short and may not happen at all. As you sleep and your brain "resets" itself throughout the night your REM sleep increases and the length of REM sleep increases. Usually the greatest amount of REM sleep occurs within an hour or two before you typically wake up. There are several important characteristics of REM sleep:

1. It is usually associated with active dreaming.

2. You are even more difficult to wake up by outside stimuli than when you are in deep slow wave sleep, and yet you usually awaken in the morning during an episode of REM sleep, not slow wave sleep.

3. Your muscle tone is exceedingly depressed, indicating strong inhibition from the excitatory centers of your brain. Interestingly, even though your bigger muscles are extremely relaxed, a few irregular muscle movements do occur, such as the muscles controlling eye movement, hence-Rapid Eye Movement sleep.

4. Your heart rate and respiratory rate become irregular which is characteristic of the dream state.

5. Your brain is highly active during REM sleep, and the overall brain metabolism may be increased as much as 20 percent. Researchers have also found that brain activity and brain waves are similar to the activity and waves when we are awake. REM sleep is also called paradoxical sleep because it is a paradox that you can still be asleep despite the increase in brain activity. REM sleep is a type of sleep in which your brain is very active. However, your brain activity is not channeled in the proper direction for you to be fully aware of your surroundings and therefore to be awake.[4]

Rest and Relaxation

Rest is essentially a period of inactivity for your mind and body. Of course our body is always working until the day we die, the so called *eternal rest*. Even in our deepest sleep our hearts continue to beat, our lungs expand and contract, and our cells are going their merry way doing the multitude of jobs that they are designed to do. But, when we rest, our body slows down from the breakneck speed that it is used to during our typical day.

As I mentioned before, rest slows down our metabolic rate or the rate at which we perform chemical reactions and expend energy. While resting, the trillions and trillions of chemical reactions our body maintains every second are reduced, thereby requiring less energy. The less energy we need also means that we don't have to breathe as hard to maintain our oxygen levels and our heart doesn't have to beat as hard to deliver the oxygen and nutrients for all of the chemical reactions. Fewer chemical reactions = less wear and tear on our cells and tissues.

The "relaxation response" is another benefit to rest. Rest has been found to decrease the levels of hormones related to stress. These "fight or flight" hormones, while crucial to our everyday survival, can have detrimental effects if they are maintained at a high level for extended periods of time. These hormones can break down tissues to be used for a quick adrenaline burst of fuel if needed, and they also divert blood flow from less critical organs and tissues. When we are involved in a stressful situation blood flow is routed away from our digestive organs and our skin; and channeled to our muscles, heart, and lungs in case we need to use them in a hurry. You may have heard the expression, "You look white as a sheet," after someone jumped out from behind a door and scared you. Blood was diverted away from your skin to supply your muscles in case you needed to make a quick get-away from the boogie man. With less blood flowing to your skin you are also less susceptible to significant damage if that tiger takes a swipe at you and happens to graze your skin.

Rest and stress, seemingly at opposite ends of the spectrum, are nonetheless closely connected. Stress, an important part of our everyday lives, has been linked to an inability to rest. If you are constantly in a state of stress, (and let's be honest, these days who isn't?) your body produces certain hormones that rev up your hard-drive and put it into overdrive. While this isn't necessarily a bad thing, prolonged periods of stress, without proper rest, can lower amounts of certain neurotransmitters which can lead to unhealthy consequences.

Now that we know how important rest is to YOU 1.0 let's take a look at some of the more common signs of not getting enough rest.

Signs You Aren't Getting Enough Rest

+ You experience waves of drowsiness during the day, such as in meetings, during lectures, or driving

+ Recent or unexplained weight gain, new research has shown that a lack of sleep can affect certain hormones which regulate metabolism and hunger

+ You rely on an alarm clock to wake you

+ You struggle to wake up and begin your activities

- Dozing off unintentionally

- Dozing off easily while reading or watching television

- You feel sleepy after a single glass of alcohol

- You feel a consistent loss of energy or alertness

- You routinely roll over and fall back to sleep when the alarm goes off in the morning

- Feeling groggy and lethargic after waking up in the morning and struggling to stay awake during the day

- Long meetings, overheated rooms, and heavy meals make you very drowsy

- Being more accident-prone or coming close to nodding off while driving

- Having a hard time concentrating on important tasks at work

- Being increasingly grumpy and irritable with your spouse and children and less able to cope even with simple problems

- Having a hard time completing simple tasks

- Weight gain resulting from the intake of sugary, high calorie foods used to try to keep you awake

- Being sick more often as a result of your immune system's inability to ward off bacteria and viruses

These signs can vary from person to person. In fact, some people can tolerate rest deprivation quite well, while others can have significant impairment with only a small amount of missed rest. Some people who are most affected by their rest habits are new mothers, late shift workers, people who travel a lot, and people in high stress jobs.

The following are some common sleep disruptors and rest busters.

Sleep disruptors/Rest busters

<u>Caffeine</u>—Caffeine can interrupt your sleep patterns even if you don't have trouble *falling* asleep.

Television in the bedroom—TV's produce light and noise, see below. Some people feel that the television helps them to fall asleep but the light and noise can interrupt your sleep cycles.

Light—Light seems to affect the production of certain chemicals in your brain which helps you to sleep during the night time and helps you to wake up during the day.

Stress—Stress affects your nervous system and chemical balance making it harder to fall asleep and harder to enter deep sleep where repair and relaxation take place.

Alcohol—Alcohol may make you feel sleepy but as the alcohol wears off it wakes you up, and you suffer from fragmented sleep for the rest of the night.

Exercise before bed—Exercise can increase your levels of adrenaline making it hard to sleep.

Noise—Noise can disrupt the sleep cycle preventing you from getting a good night's sleep.

Children/Pets—Additional items in bed with you, even cute and snuggly things, have a good chance of waking you up in the night.

Temperature—Usually being too warm rather than too cold is the main problem. Being warm is a signal for your body to wake-up, which makes it hard to remain asleep.

Why Can't Americans Rest?

It's an interesting question, we know rest is good for us yet we just can't seem to fit it into our busy schedules. What is it about Americans that makes it so hard to rest? A little history may be in order. Efficiency and restlessness may just be in our genes. Most of us have forefathers who championed the Protestant work ethic, a philosophy that looked at rest and idleness as work of the devil. "Idle hands are the devil's tools" and "Time is money" were popular sayings that encouraged Americans not to waste their time. Because of this philosophy Americans have been hard at work inventing even more time saving devices that allow us to accomplish more and more in less time. The light bulb allowed us to work well into the night. The telephone allowed us to contact others instantly instead of waiting for the postal service. Automated machines and power tools help us to create more in less time. The computer connected us to the world in an instant, including our office while sitting at home in our Lazy-Boy.

There is nothing to stop us from working 24 hours a day except our own mind and body. With all of this time saving technology some theorists 30-40 years ago postulated that our work-week would decline to 20 hours per week or less. Instead, our average work week has hovered around 40 hours per week since the 1960's. (That is hours worked in *the office or on the job*, that figure does not include time spent at home working.)

It is not only our own ingenuity and industriousness that keeps us from resting however. The very nature of our capitalist society perpetuates our "workaholic" tendencies. The more we work the more we can purchase. We are not content with the status quo. Our houses are bigger than ever before and we "can't live without" much more than our grandparents lived without. Fax machines, video games, espresso makers, air conditioning, CD players, microwaves, and dishwashers are luxury items that we can't or more appropriately WON'T live without. So, the more we work the more money we can make which equals more stuff, and more stuff means that we can do more in the limited time we have.

Our technological advances have not only created more for us to do but they have also created a culture of impatience. Computers have become faster and faster but not nearly fast enough. We can cook an entire meal in the microwave in 10 minutes or we can just as easily drive thru a McDonald's and be munching on a Big Mac within 2-3 minutes. We expect things NOW and when we don't get them we feel that we are wasting time. So how do we take a step back, catch our breath and learn to rest? That is the focus of the next chapter, read on.

References

1. Guyton, AC, Hall, JE. *Textbook of Medical Physiology.* 9th ed._Page 761. W. B. Saunders Company, Philadelphia, 1996.

2. Guyton, AC, Hall, JE. *Textbook of Medical Physiology.* 9th ed._Page 763. W. B. Saunders Company, Philadelphia, 1996.

3. Mass, JB. *Power Sleep*, Villard, New York, 1998.

4. Guyton, AC, Hall, JE. *Textbook of Medical Physiology.* 9th ed._Page 762. W. B. Saunders Company, Philadelphia, 1996.

5.0

IMPROVING REST

A good laugh and a long sleep are the best cures in the doctor's book.

Irish Proverb

Getting enough rest is just as important to YOU 1.0 as the other components of the PRIME operating system. This chapter will tell you how to get the rest you need.

Some of the benefits of getting enough rest include:

- Improved immune system function and reduced recovery time from illness
- Greater concentration and creativity
- Fewer aches and pains with reduced muscle tension
- Less risk for disease
- Better ability to learn and improved memory function
- Better job performance, satisfaction, and productivity
- Less stress and better control over the unavoidable stress in our lives.
- Lower blood pressure
- Improved social ability and positive mental attitude

Trouble Falling Asleep?

Many studies over the past few years have found that few people are free of sleep problems. A recent poll estimated that 56% of American adults have sleep problems, up from 35% in 1990. The result: over thirty-five million prescriptions for sleeping pills and over 2.5 billion dollars spent on over the counter medications. Yet, more than 33% say they get less sleep now than 5 years ago.

Sleep is critical to good health and functioning, so lack of it is a serious matter. Research suggests that the primary reason for sleep is not just rest, but more importantly…recovery. While we sleep enzymes activate protein production for repair, our immune system is activated, and our bodies get to work trying to fix the damage we managed to do during the day. All of this activity takes place as planned *if* we get the quality and quantity of sleep we need.

Here are a few tips to help you get the vital sleep you need each and every night.

10.0 Tips for sleep:

1.0 Hide the clock

Most of us wake up at night at least a few times. In fact, at the end of every cycle of REM sleep we tend to wake up to some degree. For some of us, we don't quite reach the conscious stage, we turn over and go right back to sleep. For others, we wake up more fully and become aware that we are awake. When this happens what do we do? We look to see what time it is, setting up a damaging cycle of waking up at the same time night after night. Or, we may needlessly worry about what time it is and how much sleep we have gotten already or how much more sleep we need to feel refreshed. Trust your internal alarm clock or your mechanical alarm clock to wake you when the time is right and simply try to relax until that time. Turn your clock away from you or put it out of reach and out of sight to make your sleep area a time free zone.

2.0 Lower the temperature

As we sleep our internal body temperature naturally drops slightly. This is due to the decreased energy demands and the lowered metabolism levels required while we sleep. A few hours before we wake, our body temperature gradually increases back to levels maintained while we are awake. If the room you sleep in is too warm you have a more difficult time lowering your body temperature, confusing your system to think that it should be awake. Buy an adjustable thermostat and set the temperature at a comfortable level while you sleep.

3.0 Keep kids and pets out of bed with you

They are so cute, so snuggly, and so hard to sleep with. Children and pets provide the joy that we need in our lives, but they are terrible at sharing a bed. They move, push, make noise, and kick while you are trying to recharge and re-boot so that you can give them your full attention the next day. Don't allow children or pets on the bed with you (or even in the same room if you can help it.) During the night your bed should be your sanctuary, help others to respect that, and you will sleep much better. A lazy Saturday or Sunday morning after you are already awake is a great time to catch up on your cuddling.

Fast Fact

One of the best predictors of insomnia later in life is the development of bad habits from having sleep disturbed by young children.

4.0 Go to sleep and get up at the same time every day

Human beings, and most living organisms, are creatures of habit. My black lab, Scout, has an internal tummy clock that is more accurate than my watch. She is fed every day at 6:30 PM and without fail, she will come and sit next to me waiting for dinner within 5 minutes of 6:30 every day. Just as Scout has a tummy clock, you have an internal wake/sleep clock. Altering the times when you go to sleep and get up can confuse your internal clock, resulting in poor quality and decreased quantity of sleep. If you get up at 6 AM on some days and at 10 AM on other days you confuse your body clock. When you get up at 6 AM you are tired because your internal clock tells you it isn't time to get up yet. When you get up at 10 AM the four hours between 6-10 AM aren't quality sleep because your body is wondering why you are still laying in bed when you should have been up 4 hours ago. Going to bed and getting up at the same time every day helps your body to recognize when it is supposed to rest and when it is supposed to be awake.

5.0 Reduce noise

Try to maintain a quiet zone while you sleep. Unexpected noises can startle you, wake you up, increase your heart rate, and elevate your blood pressure. Unexpected noises can come from any number of places such as emergency vehicle sirens, barking dogs, crying babies, and even an obnoxious commercial on the television. Turn the TV off, and sound proof your sleeping area as much as possible. If you are still awakened by noises at night, turn on a fan or a radio and tune it to static. You will become accustomed to the noise and it will help to drown out any other unexpected sounds.

6.0 Reduce light

Light plays an important part in our circadian rhythms of wakefulness and sleepiness. Studies have shown that light can seriously affect the quality and quantity of our sleep. Pull the shades completely shut or cover your windows with dark fabric to keep the light out of your sleep quarters. Even the light from a television can affect your sleep, so turn it off. If all else fails, a good comfortable sleep mask will do the trick.

> **Fast Fact**
> The tiny amount of light from a digital alarm clock can be enough to disrupt the sleep cycle even if you do not fully wake. The light turns off a "neural switch" in the brain, causing levels of a key sleep chemical to decline within minutes.

7.0 Buy a quality mattress

Choosing a comfortable mattress is critical to getting a good night's sleep. A mattress should provide uniform support from head to toe. If there are gaps between your body and your mattress you're not getting the full support you need. Every few months, turn your mattress clockwise or upside down so that your mattress wears evenly. If you're waking up uncomfortable, it may be time for a new mattress. There is no standard lifespan for a mattress, it simply depends upon its quality and what kind of usage it gets.

8.0 Use a good pillow

Your pillow can be your best friend at night, or your worst enemy. After spending hundreds or thousands of dollars on a mattress, don't skimp on a pillow that doesn't support your head and neck properly. A good pillow may cost as much as $100. Sounds like a lot doesn't it? Remember this however, your car probably cost you one hundred to five hundred times that, if not significantly more. A good quality pillow can last you up to 10 years. At 8 hours of sleep per night, that is 29,200 hours of use. Let's say you keep your car for 10 years, (unlikely) and drive it 2 hours per day-that is a total of 7,300 hours of use—quite a bit less isn't it? *And,* driving isn't critical to your health and well-being.

Be selective when shopping for a pillow. When lying on your side, your head and neck should be level with your mid and lower spine. When lying on your back, your head and neck should remain level with your upper back and spine. In other words, your pillow should not be so thick that it causes your head and neck to be propped up or angled sharply away from your body. Be wary of pillows that are made out of mushy foam materials. The weight of your head can displace this kind of foam, leaving little support. Choose a pillow with firm foam that supports your head. There is no such thing as a universal fit when it comes to pillows. Find one that is consistent with the shape and size of your body.

9.0 Sleep on your side or back only

Avoid sleeping on your stomach. Sleeping on your stomach forces your head to rotate at an extreme angle for extended periods of time, typically causing you to wake up in the middle of the night to change position. Sleep on your side or on your back, keeping in mind the position of your head and neck. On your side, your head and neck should be level with the rest of your spine. On your back, your pillow should support your neck maintaining the proper curvature of your cervical spine. When you correctly support your neck you help to prevent frequent "wake-ups," headaches, backaches, and general aches and pains caused by wear and tear on your vertebral column.

10.0 Eat at least 2 hours before bed time

Eating after 6 PM may interfere with sleep as your body works to digest the food you've eaten. While a large meal may make you feel tired initially after eating it, you may have problems digesting the food causing heartburn, indigestion, or gas which will keep you tossing and turning throughout the night.

In addition to sleep related problems you are more likely to gain weight if you eat close to bedtime as well. After a meal your body pumps insulin into your blood stream stimulating absorbtion of carbohydrates and conversion of those sugars into fat. Pair the realative inactivity and low calorie burning state of sleep with the high rate of insulin secretion and fat production and you have a recipe for weight gain.

Fast Fact
Anything less than five minutes to fall asleep at night means you're sleep deprived. The ideal is between 10 and 15 minutes, meaning you're still tired enough to sleep deeply, but not so exhausted you feel sleepy by day.

As we have seen, sleep and rest are separate entities. The following 5 tips will help you to improve how you rest.

5.0 Tips for Rest:

1.0 Practice deep breathing

Deep breathing has been practiced for centuries by monks, yoga masters, and natural healers. A research study performed in 2001 shows that it can be beneficial for you too. Deep, slow breathing was found to reduce the effects of the sympathetic nervous system on your heart which raises heart rate and blood pressure. Slow, deep breathing helps to saturate your blood with oxygen and increases the sensitivity of certain nerve receptors in your arteries which when stimulated help to lower blood pressure.[1]

2.0 Yoga

Yoga has been practiced in some form for thousands of years. Sanskrit documents have been found that contain yoga poses and mantras that are four thousand years old! The first book of any kind is believed to be a book about yoga. Many of the ancient poses and movements have been adapted by physical therapists and physiatrists in the 19th and 20th centuries to help them heal their patients.

Yoga can be a powerful stress buster and can help you to relax and calm your physical, emotional, and mental being. Try yoga to help you rest and relax, it works.

3.0 Eat right

Just as rest is important to health, so are the other 4 components of the PRIME operating system including your Intake. People with a healthy Intake are better able to rest. Eating a healthy diet consisting of fruits, vegetables, whole grains, poultry, and fish will provide your body the natural building blocks it needs to produce your own relaxing neurotransmitters produced in your brain and body.

Tryptophan, an amino acid found in protein and foods like turkey, helps to stimulate the release of serotonin in your brain which has a natural calming effect. Calcium, which is found in dairy products as well as leafy green vegetables also has relaxation properties. It stimulates the release of melatonin which is a natural hormone that regulates the body's reaction to light and dark, and therefore is a natural rest promoter. Calcium also seems to help to calm your neuro-muscular system which will help you to rest.

4.0 Take a 15 minute nap

If you don't have trouble falling asleep at night, a mid-afternoon nap can be quite relaxing. In fact, some researchers have found that a tendency to get sleepy during the day is a biological response even after a good night's sleep. It seems that our bodies go through a sleep cycle that occurs in the evening and again around 1-4 PM. Some scientists believe that it is a survival response passed on from our primitive ancestors to keep us out of the hot mid-day sun.[2]

Naps have been shown to reduce stress, reduce the risk of heart disease, restore alertness, increase the ability to pay attention to details, and make critical decisions.[2] Avoid naps late in the afternoon and naps longer than 30 minutes. They may inhibit your ability to fall asleep later that night.

5.0 Take time for yourself

Sometimes we get so caught up in dealing with the things we have to do that we don't take time for ourselves. If we do happen to get a few free minutes of time to rest, we cannot fully enjoy it because we are worrying about things we still have to do. If you find yourself in this situation, schedule time for yourself on your list of things to do.

Take a Saturday afternoon or an evening off from your normal hectic lifestyle and pencil in some rest time for yourself. Better yet, take a vacation, or at least a vacation day off from work or the kids. Tell the boss or get a sitter, delegate some of your responsibilities, and put your other "to-do" things on the back burner, at least for awhile. Don't worry about all of the things you could or should be doing and rest without guilt. You deserve it.

Stress and rest are intimately connected. We will cover stress in a later chapter.

References

1. Bernardi L, Porta C, Spicuzza L, Bellwon J, Spadacini G, Frey AW, Yeung LY, Sanderson JE, Pedretti R, Tramarin R. *Slow breathing increases arterial baroreflex sensitivity in patients with chronic heart failure.* Circulation. 2002 Jan 15;105(2):143-5.

2. Mass, James B. *Power Sleep*, Villard, New York 1998

6.0

INTAKE

In all the controversies over what the causes of disease might be, no one seems to have paid much attention to the factor in the environment that has the most obvious effect on any organism: food.

Michael Crawford & David Marsh,
The Driving Force: Food in Evolution and the Future

The third cornerstone for a foundation of wellness is INTAKE. Intake represents everything you put into your body or ingest. What we put into our bodies is as important as the other 4 components of the PRIME operating system. The old computer code-writers saying "Garbage in-garbage out," seems particularly appropriate for this section. This chapter will cover the importance of what we intake every day. And, because today more than ever, most of us are lucky enough (or unlucky enough!) to have an abundance of foods available at our fingertips, we will be discussing weight loss and weight management.

For the past 2000 years the human diet has changed very little. We ate meats, cheeses, whole grains, fruits and vegetables. Over the past 40 years or so however, we have seen a revolution in the way we eat. The basic foods and drink we consume have changed dramatically. And because of these changes, 4 of the top 10 causes of death in the U.S. are directly related to diets that are too high in fat, cholesterol, sugars, and too low in fiber.

In this day and age we purchase and eat fast food and delivered pizzas which, while convenient for the person on the go, are high in fat and calories. Prepackaged and pre-made meals and microwavable dinners are also high in fat and calories. Enriched flour is added to our breads and pastas, which doesn't sound so bad. The word "enriched flour" on a food label however, means that the wheat which makes the flour has been highly refined and stripped of the 11 known vitamins, 6 nutritional minerals, and essential fatty acids. Then the flour is put through a chemical process to artificially insert 4 of the lost vitamins and 1 mineral, iron. Enriched? Hardly.

In 1945, Americans drank more than four times as much milk as carbonated soft drinks. In 1997, we downed nearly two and a half times more soda than milk, almost 55 gallons per person per year.[1] Soft drink consumption in adults has increased 61 percent from 1977 to 1997. During the same time period soft drink consumption by children has increased 100 percent.

Fast Fact
Each 12 ounce can of soda has about 10 teaspoons of sugar in it. Speaking of sugar, candy consumption reached an all time high of 25 pounds per person in 1997.

In the year 2000, our caloric intake was calculated to be about 2700 calories per person per day. Compare that to our caloric intake just 30 years ago, which was estimated to be almost 20% less, or 530 calories per person per day *less,* than today. Since the turn of the century (1900), technology has grown at an unprecedented pace. New advances helped to initiate and encourage other even more exciting breakthroughs. Our diet has also changed, but towards a more discouraging direction. Increased caloric intake, and corresponding increases in average body weight, fat mass, blood pressure, and obesity, as well as reduced fruit and vegetable, fiber, and complex carbohydrate intake have turned us into a society of "point, click, and jigglers." Once again, we have sacrificed our health for speed and convenience. All is not lost however my friend, go grab an apple to munch on, and read on.

The foods we eat and the liquids we drink have many different roles in the functioning of our bodies. The primary reason we eat is to provide energy to the trillions of cells within our body for actions, building, and repair. Every heart beat, every breath, every blink of an eye, every nerve impulse, every cell division, and virtually every action our body makes, requires energy. We are living, breathing, moving power plants that produce and consume energy. You intake complex materials and break them down into their base forms such as proteins, carbohydrates, fats, vitamins, and minerals. Next, you transport these raw materials to a storage depot like your liver or fat cells, or you use them immediately to power muscles, initiate chemical reactions, or build the raw materials into more useful end products like hormones. The raw materials we don't need we store in our muscles, fat, and liver for later use; or we discard them through our kidneys and bowels. You really are pretty amazing don't you think?

Most commonly we think of eating as a way to accomplish our physiological needs for nourishment. Food is our power source, just like the electricity coming from a battery or the wall outlet is the power source for your computer. As living beings we have to eat or we will die. This is the main reason to be sure, but in our society where food is only a walk to the fridge or a short ride down to the drive-thru, we seldom NEED to eat. We typically eat breakfast, lunch, and dinner (or supper if you are from the North) whether we are hungry or not. Why do we do this? At this point it is not a survival mechanism, but more of a social activity. Eating is a great way to catch up with an old friend, interact with family, or impress your blind date with your witty banter.

In addition to being a social activity, eating also relieves stress. While we eat, and for a time after, our parasympathetic nervous system is activated helping us to digest our food. When our parasympathetic nervous system is activated it quiets our sympathetic nervous system, which mediates our stress levels or our so called "fight or flight" responses. Have you ever felt relaxed after eating a big meal? Sometimes we feel so relaxed that a nap sounds like a pretty good idea. Unfortunately your boss usually doesn't see eye to eye with you on this subject. In some societies an afternoon nap or siesta after a meal is not only socially acceptable, it is expected. Sometimes we eat things that are considered comfort food that make us feel better. These foods are usually high in fat and carbohydrates (like ice cream and chocolate) which have a high glycemic index, stimulating the release of insulin which signals your body to store excess energy. After eating, your body typically responds by going into storage mode which makes you feel more relaxed. There are many reasons why we eat. Learning to understand and identify these reasons can help you to determine whether you are eating to relieve stress, because you are with friends, or because you are truly hungry.

Major Food Categories

In order to understand how to modify and regulate our INTAKE for a strong foundation, let's take a look at the building blocks of what we are eating.

There are two major categories for the foods we eat, macronutrients and micronutrients. Macronutrients are proteins, carbohydrates, and fats. These three categories of nutrients are the sources of energy for your body and they make up the overwhelming majority of our diets. Micronutrients are other substances in food such as vitamins and minerals which regulate the functions inside and outside your cells. These substances are required in much smaller amounts, therefore they are called micronutrients.

First the macronutrients. Fat, protein, and carbohydrates are considered your fuel nutrients because they are the only substances that provide your body calories or energy. (Actually alcohol also has calories but it is usually not grouped with the other macronutrients.) A calorie is a unit of measurement that describes a unit of energy, either supplied by food or burned by your body. Scientifically, a calorie is the amount of energy required to raise the temperature of 1 gram of water 1 degree Celsius. Fat has more than twice the calories per gram (9) than the other macronutrients, and is therefore a very efficient storage unit for your body's energy. Carbohydrates and proteins each contain 4 calories per gram. (Alcohol contains 7 calories per gram.) Let's talk about fat first.

Fat

In this day and age fat is the macronutrient that we love to hate. The fact of the matter is that we need fat to survive. Fats form the cell membranes that surround every cell in your body. Fat is stored under our skin to keep us warm and it is located within muscle tissue to provide energy for them to do work. Fat also protects our internal organs and helps to absorb, transport, and store fat soluble vitamins like vitamin A, D, E, and K. Fat is so important that our bodies actually produce most of the fat we need from excess carbohydrates and proteins in our diet. The problem is that we consume too much of it! Fat helps to make things taste good. Some of the best tasting foods like, fast foods, chocolate, butter, ice cream, and cheese also have some of the highest fat content.

It is no surprise that we have evolved to enjoy the taste of foods that contain fat. Fat is the perfect energy storage unit because of its high calorie per gram ratio of energy availability. 20,000 years ago when we had to fight for every scrap of food we got, fat was a very efficient way for us to get the calories we needed to survive. We acquired a taste for foods with fat in them out of necessity. Unfortunately for most of us today, we only <u>need</u> a small amount of fat, equal to about a tablespoon of vegetable oil a day.

Typically simple fats come in two different forms: saturated and unsaturated. Saturated fats usually come from animal products and are solid at room temperature, like the fat on a steak. Saturated fats are generally thought of as the "bad" fat because they have been linked to increased cholesterol levels which promote plaque build-up in your arteries.

Unsaturated fats come from vegetables and are liquid at room temperature. Common unsaturated fats are cooking oils such as sunflower oil, olive oil, canola oil, and many others. Unsaturated fats are categorized as monounsaturated or polyunsaturated. Monounsaturated fats are typically considered the "good" type of unsaturated fatty acids because they have been shown to increase your levels of HDL (good cholesterol) and to lower levels of LDL (bad cholesterol). Monounsaturated fatty acids can be found in all of the vegetable oils but are especially abundant in olive oil, canola oil, and peanut oils.

Current recommendations for fat intake are that 30% of your calories per day should come from fat, with the majority coming from monounsaturated and polyunsaturated fatty acids. Higher intakes of dietary fat, especially saturated animal fat, have been shown to increase the risks of developing certain cancers including breast, colon, prostate, and pancreas.[2]

Protein

Protein is another macronutrient that our body cannot do without. Protein can be found in animal tissues such as beef, pork, fish, and chicken; dairy products; and in vegetables like beans and rice. Proteins are mostly broken down by your digestive system into their base components, amino acids, and then they are reassembled for the many roles that they play in your body. Proteins and amino acids help to form enzymes which speed up chemical reactions in your cells. They also help to form antibodies which your immune system regulates to help fight off disease. Proteins are also used for hormone production. Hormones regulate many different bodily functions such as your sugar absorption rate, stress response, and metabolism. Proteins are also the main components that your body uses to build and repair tissues.

Proteins are not typically used for energy, although they can be converted into fuel during periods of low carbohydrate and low fat consumption, i.e.: dieting. Just as protein can be converted into fuel, it can also be converted into fatty tissue, just like the other macronutrients if your calorie consumption exceeds your calorie burn rate.

Carbohydrates

The third category of macronutrient is carbohydrate. "Carbs" are your body's primary source of fuel. Some common carbs include bread, grain, cereal, fruits, vegetables, and sugar. Carbohydrates can be broken down into three major categories: Simple carbohydrates or sugars, complex carbohydrates or sugars, and fiber.

Simple carbohydrates are carbs that consist of one or two simple sugars like glucose, fructose, or lactose. Simple sugars are found in things like: fruits, corn syrup, honey, table sugar, maple syrup, and beer. Regardless of whatever form simple sugars are found in, they must be broken down into glucose. Glucose is the only sugar molecule that your body can use in its natural form. These simple carbohydrates are easily broken down and converted into energy by your body. Or, if energy is not needed at that particular moment, they can be stored as fat or glycogen (a stored energy molecule) to be used later.

Complex carbohydrates do not have a sweet taste like many simple carbs and are commonly referred to as starch. Starch is found in vegetables such as wheat, corn, potatoes, beans, and peas. Starches are also easily converted into energy or stored for later use.

Fiber is often considered a complex carbohydrate as well. Fiber consists of non-digestible carbohydrates and provides no energy or micronutrients to your body. It is however, essential to a healthy diet because of its unique properties. Some types of fiber bind to cholesterol in the digestive tract

> **Fast fact**
> High fiber foods should be added gradually to your diet to minimize gastrointestinal symptoms, which may include gas, cramps, and diarrhea. Excessive fiber intake may also decrease the absorption of drugs, vitamins, minerals, and other nutrients. It is generally recommended you limit your intake to 35 grams of fiber per day, although most of us struggle to reach that mark!

which then helps to lower the cholesterol level in the blood stream.[3] Fiber also adds bulk to your diet which increases bowel motility and elimination of food waste products. For people who live in countries where high-fiber diets are the norm, the average transit time for food is 24-48 hours, compared with that of the average American, whose average transit time is 72 hours or greater. Fiber and increased intestinal motility has been shown to reduce the risk of developing certain types of intestinal cancers and intestinal diverticula or polyps.[4] High intake of fiber has also been associated with a reduced risk of cancer in hormonal tissues, including the breast and ovaries.[5] Fiber is found naturally in whole grain breads and cereals, fruits and vegetables.

Micronutrients

Vitamins, minerals, antioxidants, and phytochemicals are all considered micronutrients. As stated earlier, micronutrients don't provide your body calories or direct energy but they are essential to every process in your body. They have a comparable role in your body as does the power button on your computer. Nothing happens in your body unless micronutrients are involved to get things started.

There have been 13 vitamins identified to date. Your body cannot make its own vitamins so most must be found in the food supply. The vitamins you need that are not supplied by your diet are made by "friendly" bacteria found in your own body! Each vitamin has a specific function that regulates a biochemical reaction in each cell of your body. Without them, reactions can't get started and you can't operate at peak efficiency.

Like vitamins, there are at least 15 minerals that we require in small amounts every day that are essential for minimal levels of good health. These are calcium, magnesium, phosphorus, sodium, potassium, sulfur, chlorine, iron, iodine, copper, manganese, zinc, molybdenum, selenium, and chromium. The minerals in our body make up about 5% of our total body weight. Minerals help to form structures like bones and help your blood carry oxygen. They also regulate metabolic functions, help your nerves to transmit impulses, and participate in enzyme reactions. Some of the most important minerals are calcium, phosphorus, sodium, potassium, and iron.

Antioxidants are the current media darlings in the micronutrient world. Antioxidants act like "free radical" scavengers, scooping up damaging free radicals which are produced by infections, when you burn energy, and by pollutants you may come into contact with. These free radicals are stray electrons that are produced through chemical reactions. After the reaction, the free radicals wander about looking for a place to grab on to. The problem is that they can grab on to critical structures like your DNA and cause disease, cell damage, and accelerate the aging process. Antioxidants are the antivirus programs of YOU 1.0. They capture dangerous free radicals and transform them into harmless compounds that you can delete at a later date. Some vitamins are also antioxidants like vitamin E and vitamin C. Intake of foods rich in these antioxidant compounds has been associated with a reduced risk of certain types of cancer as well as decreased frequency of other chronic health problems.

Phytochemicals are a relatively recent discovery. They are plant compounds with antioxidant properties. They are often referred to as "anti-cancer" compounds, but they seem to have a protective role in heart health and vision as well. Phytochemicals are associated with the prevention and/or treatment of at least four of the leading causes of death in the United States—cancer, diabetes, cardiovascular disease, and hypertension.[6] Currently, researchers have identified over 1000 different phytochemicals and scientists continue to discover more every day. It is estimated that there may be more than 100 different phytochemicals in just one serving of vegetables.[7] Lycopene, which is found in red tomatoes and tomato sauce is a phytochemical you may have heard of.

Below is a list of 13 common vitamins, 7 minerals, and 9 trace elements. Also listed is what they are needed for, and how you can incorporate them into your intake plan.

Vitamins

Vitamin	Needed For	Good Sources
Vitamin A (and beta-carotene)	Healthy skin, strong teeth and bones in children, maintaining resistance to infection, normal growth, cell structure, normal eyesight	Fish liver oils, liver, dairy products (vitamin A); carrots, dark-green leafy vegetables (beta-carotene)
Vitamin B-1 (thiamine)	Use of carbohydrates in the body, digestion and appetite, normal function of nervous system	Whole grains, brown rice, beans, peas, organ meats, lean pork, seeds/nuts
Vitamin B-2 (riboflavin)	Normal growth, formation of certain enzymes, cellular Normal growth, formation of certain enzymes, cellular oxidation, prevention of sores and swelling of mouth and tongue	Dairy products, meats, poultry, fish, green vegetables (broccoli, turnip greens, asparagus, spinach)
Vitamin B-6 (pyridoxine)	Use of amino acids in the body, making hemoglobin	Meats, whole grains, wheat germ, brewer's yeast
Vitamin B-12	Nervous system functions, normal development of red blood cells, production of genetic material in cells, effective use of carbohydrates and folic acid from foods	Fish, dairy products, organ meats, beef, pork, eggs
Biotin	Activities of enzymes needed to break down fatty acids in carbohydrates, ridding the body of wastes from breakdown of proteins	Nuts, whole grains, vegetables, fruits, milk, organ meats, brewer's yeast
Folic acid	Important metabolic processes in the body, growth, reproduction, production of red blood cells	Green leafy vegetables, oranges, beans, peas, rice, eggs, liver
Pantothenic acid	Production of certain hormones, activities of enzymes in the body's use of fats and carbohydrates, use of vitamins, normal growth, nervous system functions	Organ meats, eggs, whole grains, brewer's yeast
Vitamin C (ascorbic acid)	Healthy skin, bones, teeth, gums, ligaments, and blood vessels; immunity to disease; wound healing; absorption of iron from the digestive tract	Citrus and other fresh fruits, fresh vegetables
Vitamin D	Strong bones; regulation of the absorption of calcium and phosphorus from the digestive tract	Fatty fish, liver, eggs, fortified milk
Vitamin E	Normal brain function, formation of red blood cells, maintaining some enzymes, normal cellular structure, protection against pollutants	Whole grains, vegetable oils, green leafy vegetables, eggs
Vitamin K	Blood clotting	Green leafy vegetables, dairy products

Minerals

Mineral	Needed For	Good Sources
Calcium	Healthy bones and teeth, nerve conduction, muscle contraction, blood clotting, production of energy, immunity to disease	Dairy products, green leafy vegetables
Chlorine	Maintaining body's fluid and electrolyte balances, digestive juices	Table salt with iodine
Magnesium	Every major biologic process, use of glucose in the body, synthesis of nucleic acids and protein, cellular energy	Meats, fish, green vegetables, dairy products
Phosphorus	Strong bones, all cell functions, cell membranes	Dairy products, fish, meats, poultry, vegetables, eggs
Potassium	Many major biologic processes, muscle contraction, nerve impulses, synthesis of nucleic acids and protein, energy production	Fresh vegetables, fresh fruits
Sodium	Water balance in tissues	Table salt, added to foods by manufacturer
Sulfur	Sulfur-containing amino acids	Onions, garlic, eggs, meat, dairy products

Trace Elements

Trace Element	Needed For	Good Sources
Chromium	Use of sugar in the body	Whole grains, spices, meats, brewer's yeast
Copper	Hemoglobin synthesis and function; production of collagen, elastin, neurotransmitters; melanin formation	Organ meats, shellfish, nuts, fruits
Fluorine	Binding calcium in bones and teeth	Fluoridated water
Iodine	Production of energy (as part of thyroid hormones)	Seafood, iodized salt
Iron	Hemoglobin synthesis and function; enzyme actions in energy production; production of collagen, elastin, neurotransmitters	Organ meats, meat, poultry, fish
Manganese	Functions not entirely understood, but needed for optimal health	Whole grains, nuts
Molybdenum	Functions not entirely understood, but needed for optimal health; detoxification of hazardous substances	Organ meats, whole grains, green leafy vegetables, milk, beans
Selenium	Functions not entirely understood, but necessary for optimal health	Broccoli, cabbage, celery, onions, garlic, whole grains, brewer's yeast, organ meats
Zinc	Immunity and healing, good eyesight, hundreds of enzyme activities	Whole grains, brewer's yeast, fish, meats

Now that we know what our food is actually made up of let's examine how we can influence and improve our intake.

References

1. ers.usda.gov

2. Shikany J, White G, *Dietary Guidelines for Chronic Disease Prevention*, South Med J 93(12):1157-1161, 2000.

3. Todd PA, Benfield P, Goa KL, *Guar gum: a review of its pharmacological properties, and use as a dietary adjunct in hypercholesterolemia*. Drugs. 1990;39:917-928.

4. Jalili T, Wildman REC, Medeiros DM. *Nutraceutical roles of dietary fiber.* J of Nutraceuticals Functional Med Foods. 2000;2(4):19-34.

5. Shikany J, White G, *Dietary Guidelines for Chronic Disease Prevention*, South Med J 93(12):1157-1161, 2000.

6. Bloch, A. et al. 1995. *Position of the American Dietetic Association: Phytochemicals and functional foods.* JADA.95: 493-496.

7. Polk, Melanie. 1996. *Feast on Phytochemicals.* AICR newsletter. Issue 51.

7.0

IMPROVING INTAKE

When diet is wrong medicine is of no use.
When diet is correct medicine is of no need.

Ancient Ayurvedic Proverb

What can you do to ensure that your body is getting the proper fuel it needs to operate at its best? This chapter will tell you what your body needs for optimum performance, and how to modify your behavior to make sure you get it. Follow these tips and YOU 1.0 will run smoothly for years to come.

Start your day out right

Breakfast is the most important meal of the day, and yet it is the most neglected. Mornings, for most of us, are usually pretty hectic. You may be getting ready for work or school, feeding and dressing the kids, and generally organizing for the day ahead. You may feel that you simply don't have time for breakfast or that you aren't that hungry in the morning. Update this behavior and you may find that you have more energy, alertness, and you may even lose some weight simply by eating a healthy breakfast.

While sleeping, your body's metabolism slows down because of your decreased activity and the decreased need for energy. Even so, your body will burn approximately 400-500 calories while you sleep. When you awaken your metabolism increases as you become more active while preparing for the day ahead. Breakfast is an additional cue to your body to fire up its metabolism, signaling your body that your 10-12 hour "fast" since your last meal is over. Some researchers believe that eating a healthy breakfast can help you to actually lose weight and keep it off. In fact, studies have shown that eating breakfast is a characteristic common to successful weight loss maintainers and may be a factor in their success.[1] Why is this? Common sense would indicate that by skipping breakfast we are also cutting out calories, right? Not necessarily. Typically the amount of calories taken in per day between those who eat breakfast and those who don't are the same.[1]

Skipping breakfast also does not mean that your body will begin to use stored body fat for energy, therefore losing fat and weight. It only prolongs the state of starvation that your body was in while you slept, keeping your metabolic rate low. If your metabolic rate is low, you are more likely to store the food that you do eat later in the day, instead of increasing your metabolic rate and burning it for energy. Skipped meals, especially breakfast, signal your body to conserve and store energy in case it is needed later. This is a protective mechanism that the human body has learned over time. Further studies have shown that skipping breakfast is not only an ineffective way to manage weight, but that eating certain foods for breakfast, such as cereal or oatmeal, is associated with a significantly lower body mass index, compared to skipping breakfast or eating meats and/or eggs for breakfast.[2]

A nutritional breakfast has also been shown to have a positive impact on cognitive function, memory, and learning ability.[3] Consumption of a complex carbohydrate breakfast compared to a simple carbohydrate breakfast has been shown to decrease tiredness and fatigue and increase the level of fullness after eating.[4]

Water

Almost 80% of our bodies are made up of water. Water can be found in almost every cell, tissue, and physiological process in our bodies. Water helps to regulate our body temperature, carries nutrients and waste products to and from our cells, cushions our joints, and provides for our natural elasticity which makes us more resilient to everyday bumps and bruises. Next to oxygen, water is the most vital substance necessary for our survival. Here are a few updates and facts to utilize for You 1.0.

Are you drinking enough water?

Unfortunately thirst is a poor indicator for dehydration. If you wait until you are thirsty, you are probably already mildly dehydrated. You are constantly losing water every time you breathe, thru your skin, and when you use the bathroom. One measure for your hydration level is your frequency of urination. You should be visiting the bathroom approximately every 2 hours. To determine the minimum ounces of fluid needed daily calculate the following: For adults and children weighing over 100 pounds divide your weight by half. This is the number of ounces of fluid needed daily. For example, if you weigh 160 pounds your minimum fluid needs are 80 ounces or ten 8 ounce glasses during an average day. If your activity level increases, if the temperature is hot or cold, or you work or live in a dry environment (office, airplane, car/truck with the A/C on) your needs are probably higher. Children weighing less than 100 pounds have special fluid needs and this formula may not be appropriate. Remember, caffeine, alcohol, and sweetened drinks don't count because they actually contribute to dehydration.[5]

Some signs that you may not be drinking enough water include:
Nausea, headaches, dark yellow to gold colored urine or infrequent urination, constipation, kidney stones, dry lips, mouth and skin, forgetfulness, and an increased body temperature.

Download these tips into your lifestyle to make sure you are drinking enough water:
+ Measure the amount of water in your usual glass or bottle, this will give you an idea of how many servings you need.
+ Keep single-serving sized bottled water in your car, backpack, or desk.
+ Develop a hydration habit-a glass of water when you wake up, one at each meal, and one at bedtime. (If you wake up in the night to use the bathroom move this last habit to about two hours before bedtime.)

- To help the rest of the family develop a hydration habit, serve glasses of water or a pitcher of water at each meal instead of sweetened fruit drinks or soda.
- Avoid caffeine, it acts as a diuretic, (dehydrates), increases urine production, and promotes fluid loss. Also remember that soda and fruit drinks don't count when "rehydrating." Fruit drinks contain more sugar than fruit juice.
- Check your urine, it should be pale yellow in color and you should urinate every 2-3 hours during the day.

Fast facts: Water

- It is a common misconception that too much water is bad for you. With the exception of certain health conditions, your body will only use the water it needs and eliminate the rest. Water is required for good kidney function and when water intake is insufficient, the kidneys must compensate by excreting more concentrated urine which may lead to kidney stones. Under normal circumstances there is no risk associated with drinking too much water.
- During exercise lasting less than 60 minutes, cold water is the preferred beverage. Electrolyte replacement is not necessary during short term exercise, and the sugar in sports drinks provides empty calories. The cold water not only serves to rehydrate fluids lost during exercise, but it also helps to cool your core temperature which becomes elevated during exercise.
- Drinking ice cold water can help you lose weight. Water can help to curb an appetite, which will make you less hungry, allowing you to eat less in order to feel full. Ice cold water also helps to burn calories. Ice cold water (40 degrees) must be warmed up to your core body temperature (98.6 degrees) which requires your body to expend energy or burn calories. It has been estimated that in order to raise the temperature of 1 gallon of ice cold water you will burn about 200 calories.

Delete: Soda pop

Americans drank more than 15 billion gallons of soda in the year 2000. That is approximately one 12 ounce can per day for every man, woman, and child in the U.S. Fifty-six percent of 8 year olds drink soft drinks daily and a third of teenage boys drink at least 3 cans of soda pop per day. As soda becomes more popular due to increased marketing focusing on younger drinkers, we should be aware of what nutritional value soft drinks have, and what happens to our bodies when we drink them. Most sodas contain sugar, caffeine, and phosphoric acid. All of these are no problem in limited amounts for a healthy person. In large quantities, or in developing adolescents, they can have a negative impact. Numerous studies have linked soft drinks to childhood obesity, tooth decay, caffeine dependence, increased risk of diabetes, and weakened bones.

The high sugar content and low nutritional value found in each bottle of soda has been linked to obesity and tooth decay. A report by a team of Harvard researchers published in *The Lancet*, a British medical journal, presented evidence that 12 year olds who drank soft drinks regularly were more likely to be overweight than those who didn't. They also found that for each additional daily serving of soda during the 19 month study, the risk of obesity increased 1.6 times, citing that the school children consumed almost 200 more calories per day than their counterparts who didn't drink soft drinks.

Caffeine, a common stimulant, has been found to be addictive and potentially harmful for developing children and adolescents. Have you ever had a caffeine withdrawal on the weekend, maybe when you didn't get your usual cup of "Joe?" Caffeine is a mood altering drug which works on your nervous system and creates a physical dependence much like any other addictive substance. While it is certainly not as dangerous as other mood altering drugs, more research is needed to determine the exact effects caffeine has on the neurochemistry of developing brains.

Phosphoric acid is a chemical compound made up of phosphorus, hydrogen, and oxygen. Phosphoric acid has been shown in animal studies to leech minerals out of bone such as calcium, magnesium, and potassium, which makes the bone more porous, brittle, and susceptible to fracture. Phosphoric acid also dehydrates us and makes it difficult for our cells to get the water, oxygen, and nutrients they need, while at the same time making it hard for our cells to remove the metabolic waste into the extracellular fluid where it can be disposed of. The soft drink industry argues that the phosphoric acid in soda pop only contributes about 2 percent of the phosphorus in the typical U.S. diet, with a 12 ounce can of soda pop averaging about 30 milligrams. There is concern however that even a few cans of soda a day can be damaging when they are consumed during the peak bone building years of childhood and adolescence.

Another concern is the double whammy of increasing obesity in our society coupled with osteoporosis or decreased bone density. We may be unwittingly setting our children up for future health problems, years into the future, at which time switching to milk, water, or fruit juice may be too late. About osteoporosis, Dr. Jim Mertz, DC, DACBR, former president of the American Chiropractic Association says, "I think that osteoporosis is a childhood condition with adult ramifications. In childhood, you're building that bony structure. But today's children sit behind computers or in front of the TV instead of running around outside-playing and participating in plenty of weight bearing activities."[6] Evidence of this trend came from a Mayo Clinic study published in the Journal of the American Medical Association in the summer of 2003. The study reports that from 1969 to 2001, the rate of forearm fractures rose 56% for girls and 32% for boys. Sundeep Khosla MD, a Mayo Clinic endocrinologist and lead author of the study says that the reasons for the increase in bone fractures is not explained but that, "dietary factors, such as increased soft drink consumption, decreased milk consumption, or changing patterns of physical activity" may have impaired our children's bone-mass development.[6]

Fruits and Vegetables

Countless studies have been performed validating the importance of getting enough fruits and vegetables in your diet. The FDA, The American Heart Association, and The National Cancer Institute recommend at least 5-9 <u>different</u> servings of fruits and vegetables per day, and that number seems to be rising. Many countries are now promoting a 10 & 10 program advocating eating 10 different fruits and 10 different vegetables a day!

Fruits and vegetables in the right quantities contain almost all of the vitamins and minerals that your body needs. For those of you who cringe at the thought of eating 5-9 servings of fruits and veggies per day consider this: 1 serving is equal to ½ a cup. Add some

> **Fast Fact: Fruits/Veggies**
> Almost every fruit and vegetable has about 80% water content. The same water content that YOU have. Hmmmm, interesting huh?

sliced bananas, strawberries or blueberries to your morning cereal with a glass of fresh orange juice and you are almost halfway there! Add some carrot sticks, an apple, or fresh broccoli for a snack, eat a salad with your lunch and eat another vegetable with your dinner and you have made it!

Eat your colors

A fun and easy way to add some color into your life and incorporate produce into you and your family's diet is to "eat your colors." Colorful fruits and vegetables contain a tremendous amount of phytochemicals, which protect the plants from sunlight, bad weather, and insects. Not only are these phytochemicals good for the plants but they are good for us as well! More than 1000 different phytochemicals have been identified as components of food, and many more phytochemicals continue to be discovered every day. It is estimated that there may be more than 100 different phytochemicals in just one serving of vegetables.[7]

Evidence has shown that populations that eat more fruit and vegetable produce have lower rates of chronic diseases. Some scientists believe that phytochemicals play a significant role in protecting our bodies from certain diseases. Phytochemicals are responsible for the color pigments that plants produce. For example, the substance that makes a blueberry blue, anthocyanin, has antioxidant properties that can be a powerful cancer inhibitor. Lycopene, the phytochemical that makes tomatoes red, is also an antioxidant that has been linked to lower rates of certain cancers as well as decreased rates of heart disease.

Unfortunately, research has shown that the top produce items that Americans are eating are the following: #1 French fries, #2 other potato products, #3 iceberg lettuce. Not exactly a phytochemical and pigment power-packed group. David Heber, author of *What Color Is Your Diet?* (Regan Books), has divided fruits and vegetables into the "seven colors of health." Heber recommends incorporating foods with a wide range of colors into your daily routine from the following groups:

Red

Tomatoes and tomato products such as juice, soups, sauces and ketchup; pink grapefruit, pink grapefruit juice, watermelon. These foods contain lycopene, which studies have shown reduces the risk of several types of cancer, including prostate cancer.

Red-Purple

Grapes, grape juice, red wine, prunes, cranberries, blueberries, blackberries and strawberries. These foods contain anthocyanins, powerful antioxidants that may have a beneficial effect on the heart by inhibiting the formation of blood clots. They may also defend against carcinogens.

Orange

Carrots, mangoes, pumpkin, winter squash, sweet potatoes, apricots, cantaloupe. These contain beta carotene, which improves communication between cells, helping them fight the spread of cancer.

Orange-Yellow

Oranges, orange juice, tangerines, yellow grapefruit, peaches, lemons, limes, papayas, pineapples, nectarines. These fruits are all high in vitamin C, a powerful antioxidant that helps protect cells.

Yellow-Green

Collard, Spinach, mustard and turnip greens; yellow corn, green beans, green peas, avocado, honeydew melon. These contain lutein, which protects the retina from radiation, reducing the risk of macular degeneration—the primary preventable cause of premature blindness in the United States.

Green

Broccoli, brussel sprouts, any type of cabbage, kale, cauliflower, watercress. These contain sulforaphane, isothiocyanate and idoles, phytochemicals that enhance the breakdown and excretion of cancer-causing compounds in the liver.

Fast Fact: Guava
Green skinned with white to pink meat, some scientists have dubbed the guava "Nature's Most Nutritious Fruit."

White-Green

Garlic, onions, chives, leeks, green onions, shallots. These alliums contain sulfur compounds that protect DNA. Other white-green fruits and vegetables, including asparagus, pears, artichokes, endive, mushrooms, celery and white wine, are rich in flavonoids—antioxidants that protect cell membranes.

The next time you are at the supermarket, see how many different colors of produce you can put into your shopping cart. Or better yet, let your children help you pick your colors so that they can sample and try different types of fruits and vegetables, some of which they may have never tried before.

> **Fast Fact:** A recent study published in the *Journal of the Science of Food and Agriculture* found that the best way to get the most health-promoting antioxidants from fresh vegetables was to eat them raw. If raw isn't your thing, the next best way to prepare vegetables is to steam them. They found that steamed broccoli lost only 6% of three major categories of antioxidants while microwaving the broccoli produced a loss of 86% of the same antioxidants.

Multi-vitamins

For most people there is nothing wrong with taking a daily multi-vitamin. According to some research, there isn't anything necessarily right about taking one either. Multi-vitamins are typically synthetic blends of the basic vitamins and minerals that current research has determined are good for you. The problem with multivitamins is that they are synthetic combinations of 20-50 different nutrients which may or may not work in conjunction with each other. The best, and oldest, way to get your essential nutrients is to eat them.

The human diet has remained relatively unchanged for thousands of years, until very recently. We evolved according to what we ate. 5000 years ago when your ancestors ate a tomato they benefited from the same 20,000 or so different chemicals found in most vine-ripened tomatoes today. One recently popular substance, Lycopene, is an example of only one of the tomato's chemical compounds which has been discovered and named. There are thousands more which are awaiting classification and naming. The data is still out on whether or not lycopene is *THE* miracle substance in tomatoes or whether it is a combination of substances which gives the tomato its healthy nutritional value. Most likely it is the synergistic quality of these chemicals working together that produce the beneficial effects of phytochemicals.

Think of it this way. Water is made up of H_2O. Which of the two elements that make up water puts out fire? Think about it for a minute. Hydrogen is highly explosive as evidenced by the Hindenburg disaster. Oxygen is equally flammable. The answer is that neither element alone will put out a fire. They must be found in the right combinations and proportions to work a certain way. The same holds true for substances we have been ingesting for thousands of years.

We didn't evolve into the magnificent species we are today by eating mega-doses of vitamin C or by squeezing the lycopene out of tomatoes and discarding the other thousands of nutrients. Simply put, unless you have a nutrient deficiency, for optimal performance you need ALL of the nutrients and the synergy they provide, found only in natural foods. So instead of relying on multi-vitamins to get your nutrients, try to eat them instead.

Delete: Fast food

I don't think a lengthy discussion is needed here is it? Fat laden burgers, fried fries, fast food tacos, etc. should not be your main fuel source. You are a finely tuned machine that needs premium fuel to operate at your best.

> **Juice Plus+ ®fast facts:**
> Juice Plus+® is a whole food supplement, made from a variety of nutritious fruits and vegetables, not a highly processed, highly fragmented vitamin or mineral supplement. Juice Plus+® is made from the freshest, highest quality fruits and vegetables which are juiced to extract their nutritional essence, and then reduced to a powder form. Because of this process Juice Plus+® provides not only a wide variety of naturally-occurring vitamins and minerals, but also the phytochemicals, antioxidants, active enzymes, chlorophyll, and other nutrients-even the fiber-found in the fresh, raw fruits and vegetables it's made from. For more information about Juice Plus+ ® visit their website at www.juiceplus.com.

O.K...What else can I eat?

In 1992 the USDA devised a food pyramid which is based on what foods Americans eat, what nutrients are in these foods, and how to make the best choices. In the last several years this "holy grail" of food guides, which is taught to everyone including school children, has come under fire. Some nutrition experts believe that it should distinguish between good fats and bad fats, and that eating 11 servings of breads and carbohydrates is too simplistic and overlooks the fact that *types* of carbohydrates are important.[8] **Newer recommendations by Walter** Willett, chairman of the department of nutrition at Harvard School of Public Health, focus more on eating whole grain foods, vegetables, fruits, and plant oils while reducing intake of red meats, butter, white rice and bread, pastas, sweets, and potatoes which are highly processed and cause blood sugar levels to spike.

Current research suggests limiting saturated fats and trans fats found in fatty meats and whole milk, and found in solid form such as vegetable shortenings and margarine. Other fats such as monounsaturated and polyunsaturated, which are usually found in liquid form like olive oil and other vegetable oils, nuts, fish, and whole grains, are thought to be good for you and your heart.

The carbohydrates that we consume should come from whole grains such as wheat, oats, brown rice, and beans. Fruits and vegetables also contain carbohydrates as well as fiber, vitamins, and minerals which are essential to your well-being. These foods help to keep your blood sugar levels on an even keel and also help you to feel full longer.

Protein should come from beans, fish, nuts, and chicken which are less fatty than red meats and contain important omega-3 fatty acids.

While no single nutrition plan is right for everyone most experts agree that a varied diet which includes a mix of the important elements of food is the base for a healthy diet. For an individualized diet plan or for more advice on input, seek counseling from a certified nutritionist.

Snacks

Try to limit your intake of simple sugars and refined carbohydrates found in candies, cookies, and crackers. These types of foods raise your blood sugar levels very quickly after eating them, which can cause your insulin levels and blood sugar levels to dip and spike erratically. This in turn can cause short bursts of energy followed by periods of depressed energy levels and tiredness. Try to maintain your blood sugar levels at an even level by eating snacks with a low glycemic index such as fruits and vegetables, protein bars, nuts. Don't forget that it is not only what you snack on but how much you eat that also contributes to blood sugar levels and weight loss or weight maintenance.

7.5

WEIGHT LOSS

The good Lord gave you a body that can stand most anything.
It's your mind you have to convince.

Vince Lombardi

No discussion about intake and nutrition would be complete without mentioning weight loss. First things first. Losing weight is hard. It is estimated that more than half of all American adults, up to 65%, are overweight or obese. According to the National Center for Health Statistics, an astounding 62 percent of adult Americans were overweight in 2000, up from 46 percent in 1980. Twenty-seven percent of adults were so far overweight that they were classified as obese (at least 30 pounds above their healthy weight)–twice the percentage classified as such in 1960. Alarmingly, an upward trend in obesity is also occurring in U.S. children. Dietary intake of calories in the year 2000 for the average American was estimated at just under 2,700 calories per person per day. The USDA's Economic Research Service data calculates that average daily calorie intake increased by 24.5 percent, or about 530 calories, between 1970 and 2000.[9]

As a nation, millions of us struggle with weight problems everyday. Weight related health conditions account for 300,000 deaths annually, second only to smoking as a preventable cause of death.[10] Most leading causes of adult death in developed nations are influenced by diet, including coronary heart disease, cancer, and stroke. Other diseases which contribute to the leading causes of death including hypertension, diabetes mellitus, obesity, and osteoporosis, are also closely linked with dietary intake, as a cause of the disease or an exacerbating factor.[11] One report on the association between diet and disease by Doll and Peto estimated that at least 35% of cancer deaths might be attributable to diet.[12] These sobering statistics would make almost anyone slightly overweight to want to shed a few pounds. Unfortunately many of us don't know how, have tried before and have gained the weight right back, or have set lofty goals that we were unable to meet. The good news is that there is growing evidence that suggests that even relatively small losses in weight (i.e. 10% of body weight) can mean significant improvements in health and well being.[13]

There are virtually thousands of books and programs available that claim to have the secret for weight loss made easy. A lot of these books and programs offer valuable tips and advice on how to lose weight safely and keep it off. Unfortunately many of these books offer nothing but a chance for the author to make a few bucks.

Weight loss is difficult at best and the most effective way to accomplish it varies from individual to individual. The only universal truth that most researchers agree on is that if you burn more calories than you consume, you will lose weight. Unfortunately for most authors (myself included), this concept is too simple to write an entire book about. It is not a secret formula or a trademarked diet plan but a basic fact of physiology.

The most widely recommended weight control diets are based on considerable evidence about effective and safe food consumption patterns. These diets specifically recommend increasing intake of vegetables, fruits, fiber, complex carbohydrates, and low fat dairy, while decreasing consumption of high calorie products that contain a lot of fat or simple sugars.

If you are trying to lose weight and have set goals for yourself, do it safely and plan to lose weight gradually. A weight loss of one-half to 2 pounds a week is usually safe, according to the Dietary Guidelines for Americans. This can be achieved by decreasing the calories eaten or increasing the calories used by 250 to 1,000 calories per day, depending on current calorie intake. Some people with serious health problems due to obesity may lose weight more rapidly under a doctor's supervision. If you plan to lose more than 15 to 20 pounds, have any health problems, or take medication on a regular basis, a doctor should evaluate you before you begin a weight-loss program.

One important thing to remember is that health is a process and not an event. In other words, if you are attempting to lose weight, expect set-backs. Weight regain, while discouraging, should not be viewed as failure. Use the set back to re-evaluate your daily choices and overall lifestyle options to prevent larger weight gains. All too often we initiate a work-out plan or a diet and we miss a couple of 6:30 AM workouts. Or we enjoy a second helping of dessert and we say to ourselves, "Well, there went my diet." Or, "I guess I just don't have what it takes to work out" and we give up. Sure, we might get on a kick in another month or two, which lasts a few weeks or a few months if we're good, until we eventually slip up again. By this time you may have entered a depressing cycle of ups and downs until you wear out. STOP IT! From now on when you miss a workout or a few workouts, or you indulge your sweet tooth on occasion, don't think of it as a system failure where you must completely shut down and start all over. Instead think of it as a minor glitch. Tell yourself, "No big deal, all I have to do is re-boot ME 1.0 and everything will be fine."

Another important concept to remember is that change takes time for YOU version 1.0. You didn't gain your extra pounds in 1 day (thank God), 1 week, or even 1 month. It is more likely that you have gained weight gradually over a considerable period of time. A little time and a little effort will be required to take it off. Set realistic goals within a realistic time frame, keep a positive attitude and you will be amazed at the results.

A great website to check out is the National Heart, Lung, and Blood Institute web page at: www.nhlbi.nih.gov. Here you can find information, interactive questionnaires on risks, guides to physical activity and behavior change, smart shopping tips, healthly recipes, and more help on weight control. The following are some helpful tips for you to download and save as you work towards a lean and mean YOU 1.0.

Tips and Info to help you lose and maintain your weight

Keep a Journal

Keeping a daily journal of what you consume can be a simple and valuable tool in measuring your intake. Simply write down everything you eat or drink for 3 days. You may be surprised at what you are absent-mindedly snacking on throughout the day. You may want to keep a journal for a longer period of time if you are initiating a weight loss program. It is important to remember to write down *everything* that you eat or drink. Take notes if you are away from your journal so that you can record it accurately later. Then at the end of the day or week, calculate how many calories you consumed and in what form, carbs, proteins, fat, fiber, etc. Don't be discouraged if you discover that you don't eat as healthfully as you thought. This task is meant to make you analyze what you intake, so that you can make the appropriate changes.

How to read a label

All foods and beverages sold in the U.S. are required by law to display a nutrition label and an ingredient list by the Food and Drug Administration. Learn what is on the label and how to read it and you can gain some valuable information about what you are eating and drinking. Some of the more common terms you will find on a nutrition label include: Serving size-This is the amount that the rest of the information (calories, carbohydrates, vitamins and minerals, etc.) is based on. Similar food products tend to have similar serving sizes which makes it easier to compare foods. For easy tips to remember portion sizes see the "What is a portion box?" below.

Calories-The calories listed are per serving. Remember that fat contains 9 calories per gram, protein and carbohydrates contain 4 calories per gram, and alcohol contains 7 calories per gram. You should be able to add up the grams of protein

Upload Now:
Control your portions to reduce your calorie intake. Order off of the children's menu or choose an appetizer for your main dish, they are usually smaller portions with fewer calories and they typically cost less. Split a dessert, if you need something sweet after dinner offer to split a dessert with someone. You will usually find someone who is more than happy to split dessert with you. When you order a sandwich ask for only half, or plan on eating only half and wrap up the rest for lunch tomorrow.

and carbohydrates and multiply by 4 and multiply the fat grams by 9 to come up with the total amount of calories per serving (In a non-alcoholic product). The manufacturers are allowed to round the numbers on a nutrition label so if you are off by a small amount in your own calculations that is acceptable.

In our non-metric society it is sometimes hard to figure out what a gram is. Remember this, 4 grams of sugar=about 1 teaspoon of sugar. So the next time you pick up that can of soda or that juice box or flavored yogurt, divide the grams of sugar by 4. That will give you the amount of sugar in teaspoons that the product contains.

% Daily Value (formerly the RDA or recommended daily allowance)–This percentage is usually based on a 2000 calorie diet. This number is helpful when comparing similar foods to see how they may differ from one another.

Vitamins and Minerals-Earlier we talked about the many different vitamins and minerals that your body needs to operate at peak efficiency. By law, food manufacturers are only required to list two vitamins, A and C, and two minerals, calcium and iron, on a food label. Some companies will list other vitamins and minerals on their nutrition label, but that is on a voluntary basis.

What is a portion?

Portion sizes are important when you are trying to calculate calories and other significant quantities of macro and micronutrients. As our appetites have increased in this country, so have portion sizes in popular restaurants. Here are some common ways to determine what is typically considered a portion.

½ cup of ice cream is about the size of a tennis ball

1 teaspoon of butter, peanut butter, or sour cream is about the size of the tip of your thumb, from the joint to the tip.

1 ounce of candy or nuts equals about one small handful.

1 cup of mashed potatoes or vegetables is about the size of your fist.

1 once of cheese is about the size of four stacked dice.

3 ounces of meat is about the size of a deck of cards.

A medium piece of fruit is about the size of a tennis ball.

Low carbohydrate diets

No discussion about nutrition would be complete without mentioning the low carbohydrate diet craze that has swept the country in the past few years. High protein diet plans are being hailed as the best method ever to shed unwanted pounds. Evidence that consumers are buying the concept are readily apparent. Sales of bacon, lunch meat, and cheese have risen while sales of carbs such as white bread, pasta, and cookies have fallen. A multitude of new "low-carb" products and even specialty "low-carb" stores have appeared seemingly overnight. (They seem to disappear almost as quickly.)

These diets have many names but are essentially very similar. Most advocate a low carbohydrate diet while substituting protein or fat for carbs. The "hook" for these diets is that you can supposedly still eat as much protein and fat as you want, as long as you limit your carbohydrate intake, and never go hungry. With these programs, initial weight loss does occur, as evidenced by the popularity of these diets. The research is still out however on the safety of long term high protein/low carb diets and whether or not these diets can help someone to maintain weight once it has been successfully lost. It is important to understand that no scientific evidence supports the claim that high-protein diets enable people to maintain their initial weight loss. In general, quick weight-loss diets don't work for most people.

Under normal dietary conditions your body primarily uses carbohydrates for fuel. When carbohydrate consumption is restricted your body turns to other sources of fuel such as fat and muscle or protein. This potentially dangerous metabolic change is called ketosis. A person in ketosis is getting energy from ketones, little carbon fragments that are the fuel created by the breakdown of fat storage. A high protein/low carbohydrate diet can cause a number of health problems such as: high cholesterol which has been linked to an increased risk of developing heart disease and cancer; kidney failure and kidney stones; gout; organ failure; and osteoporosis. Ketosis can be especially risky for people with diabetes because it can speed the progression of diabetic renal disease.[14] Ketosis can also dull a person's appetite, cause nausea, and bad breath. Ketosis is prevented by eating at least 100 grams of carbohydrates a day.[15]

Upload Now...

A potential problem with low carb products being offered to consumers today is that currently there are no FDA regulations on what can be called "low-carb" and what can't. This means that a food manufacturer can essentially call a product "low-carb" when in fact it may not have a low carbohydrate content at all. Always read the nutritional label and check for carbohydrate content, calorie count, and portion size, (1 cookie shouldn't equal 3 portions, etc.) And remember, a calorie is a calorie, no matter where it comes from.

> **Fast fact/Important update:**
> High protein diets should be initiated with caution especially in adolescents and women of menopausal age and older. High protein consumption has been linked to an increase in urinary calcium excretion which may lead to osteoporosis and an increased potential for broken bones. Simply increasing your protein consumption from 60 grams per day to 100 grams per day (a moderate amount in the typical US diet) doubles the amount of calcium required by the average person per day.[16]

Exercise

If you would like to lose weight, incorporate an exercise program into your routine. Many studies have shown that dieting alone is an ineffective way to lose weight. In fact, one researcher said that you would be more likely to recover from almost any form of cancer than you would be to succeed, permanently, with weight loss from dieting alone.[17] For more information on exercise see chapter 10.0.

Delete: Smoking

We all know about the risks of smoking. If you still can't quite give it up for yourself, do it for someone you love. A new study found that childhood exposure to smoke may lead to back pain later in life. One explanation, say the researchers, could be the effects of the smoke on the developing spine. In several studies, smoking has been associated with the occurrence of spinal pain, mostly low back pain, but also neck pain and prolapsed cervical intervertebral discs, says the report in the European Journal of Public Health.[18]

Delete emotional eating

Emotional eating is the #1 reason people can't lose weight and keep it off. Five of the most common reasons we emotionally eat are:

1. Hopelessness
You say to yourself, it doesn't really matter anyways. Nothing will change, so why should I worry about my health. Besides, eating makes me feel better so why not?

2. Lack of Control

You feel that you have no control over any aspect of your life except for what you eat. You can eat whenever and whatever you want and no one can stop you. This gives you a feeling that at least you can control one aspect of your life.

3. Anger

When you are angry with yourself or with someone else, you cover up your feelings with food rather than confronting the person you are angry with.

4. Boredom

You feel that there is nothing to do and nowhere to go. You don't have anything better to do so why not enjoy yourself a little.

5. Feeling Unappreciated

Maybe no one has noticed your recent accomplishment and you are feeling underappreciated. You want to treat yourself, and since no one else will, you decide to binge eat.

So how do you conquer those times when all you want is a brownie or a hot fudge sundae? Practice stress relief exercise, create a list of positive/healthy things you can do that satisfy your cravings for self-nurturing. Some positive activities include: taking a bubble bath, getting a massage, or going shopping. If money is tight create a list of free things that you can do. Some examples to help you get started are: Go for a walk, call a friend you haven't spoken to in a while, play a game, or enjoy quiet time by yourself.

Another way to help curb emotional eating is to rate your level of hunger. You can use a 1-5 scale with 1=physically hungry, 2,3=satisfied and comfortable, 4=full, 5=uncomfortably full. Use the scale to help you determine when you truly need to eat, not just when you feel like eating.

References

1. Wyatt HR, Grunwald GK, Mosca CL, Klem ML, Wing RR, Hill JO, *Long Term weight loss and breakfast in subjects in the National Weight Control Registry.* Obes Res 2002 Feb;10(2):78-82.

2. Cho, S., Dietrich M, Brown CJ, Clark CA, Block G, *The effect of breakfast type on total daily energy intake and body mass index: results from the Third National Health and Nutrition Survey.* J Am Coll Nutr. 2003, Aug;22:296-302.

3. Benton D, Parker PY. *Breakfast, Blood Glucose, and Cognition.* Am J Clin Nut 1998 Apr;67(4):772S-778S.

4. Pasman WJ, Blokdijk VM, Bertina FM, Hopman WP, Hendriks HF *Effect of two breakfasts, different in carbohydrate composition, on hunger and satiety and mood in healthy men.* Int J Obes Relat Metab Disord. 2003 Jun;27(6): 663-8.

5. Suntory Water Group, Inc. 2001, www.water.com

6. Journal of the American Chiropractic Association. Volume 41 (5), May 2004, page 9-10.

7. Polk, Melanie. 1996. *Feast on Phytochemicals.* AICR newsletter. Issue 51.

8. *New shape of the food pyramid.* By Nanci Hellmich, USA TODAY 07/26/2001.

9. USDA Agricultural Fact Book, 2001-2002.

10. McGinnis JM, Foege WH: *Actual causes of death in the United States.* JAMA 1993;270(18):2207-2212

11. Shikany, JM, *Dietary Guidelines for Chronic Disease Prevention.* Southern Medical Association Journal, 93(12):1157-1161, 2000

12. Doll R, Peto R: *The causes of cancer: quantitative estimates of avoidable risks of cancer in the United States today.* J Natl Cancer Inst 1981; 66:1191-1308.

13. National Heart, Lung, and Blood Institute, Obesity Education Initiative Expert Panel: *The Practical Guide: Identification, Evaluation and Treatment of*

Overweight and Obesity in Adults. National Institutes of Health publication No. 00-4084, Rockville, MD, October 2000.

14. *U.S. Food and Drug Administration* FDA Consumer magazine January-February 2002 Losing Weight: More Than Counting Calories By Linda Bren Publication No. (FDA) 03-1303

15. Reviewed by the Cleveland Clinic Department of Nutritional Therapy, edited by Charlotte E. Grayson, MD August 2003.

16. Nordin BE, Need AG, Steurer T, et al: *Nutrition, osteoporosis, and aging.* Ann NY Acad Sci 1998; 854:336-351.

17. Brownell KD, *Obesity=Understanding and treating a serious, prevalent and refractory disorder.* J of Consulting and Clinical Psyc. 50(1982):820-840.

18. Dobson, R, *Childhood Exposure to Smoke May Lead to Back Pain.* EJPH 2004:14; 296-300.

8.0

MIND

A strong positive attitude will create more miracles than any wonder drug.

Patricia Neal

Almost everyone has the same parts and pieces that make up their general anatomy. We all have a heart, muscles, a stomach, a kidney or two, a brain, a spinal cord, and many other "parts." What is profoundly different, no matter how alike we may seem and no matter how identical some twins are, is our mind. Your mind separates you from every person that has, is, or will walk on this earth. The human mind is a complex and fascinating marvel of different cells and chemicals processing information, emotions, and experiences all working in harmony to make YOU 1.0...well, you.

From the moment we are born we are constantly creating new connections and pathways for the cells in our nervous system. It is this constant monitoring and rearrangement of connections among our nerves that enable us to learn and to experience the world around us. How we relate to certain sights, sounds, textures, smells, and tastes is determined by thousands of different circumstances that are unique to each one of us. Your mind, without a doubt, is your most valuable asset.

First, let's explore your nervous system for a moment, the place your mind calls home. Your nervous system is composed of nerve cells which are found in your spinal cord, brain, and virtually everywhere in between. Gray's Anatomy defines the nervous system as the master system which controls and coordinates all of the organs and structures in the body and relates the individual to his/her environment.[1] Your nervous system or mind is essentially your operating system, running all of the other important processes that your body requires for life. Your nervous system monitors your heart rate and breathing to insure that you are getting enough oxygen to all of your cells. It also regulates your digestion and elimination of waste products. As mentioned earlier, your nervous system also relates you to your environment through your five senses. These are all very important jobs so it takes a sophisticated system to control all of this activity.

Fast facts, your nervous system

There are 100 billion nerve cells packed into every human head, as many as there are stars in the Milky Way. Each one of the 100 billion nerve cells in the brain is connected with up to 1 hundred thousand others, in fact, if you wanted to count each nerve connection in the brain cortex-the outer layer only-at the rate of one per second you would have to set aside about 76 thousand years! Each nerve cell is capable of making many more connections. Some scientists believe that new connections are made each time we experience or learn something new. In theory, the number of interconnections between each brain cell can be an infinite number.(Think of a 1 followed by 6 ½ million miles of zeros all this big '0'.)

The brain makes up about 2% of your body weight but accounts for up to 20% of your body's energy needs. Some researchers have suggested that at any given moment there are between 100,000 and 1,000,000 different chemical reactions taking place in your brain. Finally, if you need further proof at how astounding you are: a super computer working at 400 million calculations per second would take one hundred years to accomplish what your brain can do in one minute.[2] How's that for YOU 1.0?

Just as the other aspects of the YOU 1.0 operating system can malfunction or not be up-to-date, your mind, as amazing as it is, may need some tweaking. Depression, anxiety, and other mood disorders seem to be at an all time high in this country. Terrorism, job cuts, the economy, even something as mundane as a traffic jam can trigger unwanted feelings and emotions. While it would be simple minded and incorrect to say that many of the mental disorders we cope with are the result of outside influences, one thing that most researchers agree on is that stress plays a major role in determining our emotional health. That being said, let's take a look at stress.

Stress

Stress is difficult to define because it means different things to different people. Simply put, stress is the way you react to any demand that requires you to adjust or respond. When you feel stressed your body releases certain chemicals to help you react to the stressful situation. These substances increase blood pressure, heart rate, respiration, metabolism, and blood flow to your muscles. The "fight or flight" response is triggered and your body releases epinephrine, norepinephrine, ACTH (adrenocorticotropin hormone), and TSH (thyroid stimulating hormone) all of which help to increase your reaction time, heighten your awareness, increase metabolism and energy production, and increase blood flow to vital organs and muscles. Just what you need when you are in a stressful situation like running from a fire or when you are being chased by an angry dog. Once the situation is over, the body stops releasing these chemicals and sends out more relaxing substances such as acetylcholine to help calm us down.

Thousands of years ago these responses to stress were vital to human survival, and they still are in some situations today. The caveman who reacted the best to the stressful situation may have been the only one to survive and pass his/her genes on to the next generation. These primitive stress adaptations of our ancestors have carried over to us today. Thankfully most of us are not put into daily life or death situations like our caveman ancestors. We are however, probably put into more "non-emergency" stressful situations more often than our caveman relatives.

Our caveman ancestors probably had more of a healthy ON/OFF method of reacting to stressful situations. When there was a threat to their safety, the stress response was on. When the threat was removed, the stress response turned off, much like turning on and off a television set. In our society stress seems to be in a constant state of on. Like the television, stress is usually on for most of us to some degree. It changes like the background noise of a TV, peaking at certain times and ebbing at others. Somewhat like when the obnoxious car salesman comes on the television screen shouting about his great new deals while you are watching relaxing coverage of a golf tournament. Today stress can be caused by any number of things, but the same chemical cascade and response is triggered. Some of the more common causes of stress include:

+ Project deadlines
+ Poor diet
+ Missed appointments
+ Marital problems
+ Not enough sleep
+ Health problems
+ Financial difficulties
+ Death
+ Crowds
+ Moving
+ Retirement
+ Pregnancy
+ Legal Problems

Even with all of our technological superiority over our ancestors we have become a society that is "Stressed Out" with chronic stress syndromes. We become "stressed" by non-life threatening situations that we have no control over like traffic jams and missed appointments. In these situations the stress response has no useful purpose. It simply adds to the wear and tear on our bodies.

When we are bombarded with stressful situations our bodies automatically produce the stress hormones mentioned earlier. If we are in a constant state of stress, we may produce and sustain abnormally high levels of epinephrine, norepinephrine, and cortisol. The physical and mental toll this takes on your body can be subtle, building over time. Or the symptoms can be quite large and overwhelming if you are unable to recognize them and respond to them in a positive way. Some recent reports state that stress, (physical, mental, postural, emotional) can be related directly to 80% of the diseases known to man.

Stress Warning Signs

The first thing we must remember is that each one of us responds differently to stressful situations. Some people may enjoy a high risk/high reward type of job or a major change like moving, while others may find it too much to bear, or overwhelming. Some people may enjoy the solitude of sitting in a traffic jam while others may find it too much too take. Most of our stress comes from common everyday activities and not life changing events. Confrontations, too much to do, and the pressure of living in a fast-paced society can all contribute to stress. As mentioned earlier, stress is not necessarily a bad thing, but when you are constantly responding to stressful situations without taking appropriate measures to reduce the physical, mental, and emotional effects, you are threatening your health and well-being.

Stress can cause physical, emotional, and behavioral disorders which can affect your health, vitality, and peace-of-mind, as well as personal and professional relationships. Too much stress can cause relatively minor illnesses like insomnia, backaches, or headaches. Too much stress and the inability to control it can also contribute to potentially life-threatening diseases like high-blood pressure and heart disease.[3]

If you are not sure about what is causing your stress it may be helpful to know some of the warning signs of stress. Once you can identify the warning signs it may make it easier to recognize how you or a loved one's body responds to stress and then you can take steps to try and help reduce it.

Your body sends out physical, emotional, and behavioral warning signs of stress.
Physical signs of stress
Stooped posture
Sweaty palms
Chronic fatigue
Weight gain or loss
Physical symptoms that your doctor cannot attribute to another condition
Emotional signs of stress
Sleep disruption
Anxiety
Anger
Inability to concentrate

Unproductive worry
Sadness
Frequent mood swings
Behavioral signs of stress
Over-reacting
Using alcohol or drugs
Acting on impulse
Withdrawing from relationships
Changing jobs often
Feeling agitated most of the time

In the next chapter we will discuss how to deal with stress and how to improve the mind of YOU 1.0.

*NOTE: It is not the purpose nor intent of this book to diagnose or treat mental disorders. If you or someone you know is suffering with a mental condition please seek the advice of a qualified professional immediately.

References

1. Goss,Charles M *Gray's Anatomy, 29th Ed.* Williams & Wilkins 1973, p.4.

2. *Biophysics of Computation. Information Processing in Single Neurons*, New York: Oxford Univ. Press, 1999. AND Bear, M.F., Connors, B.W. and Pradiso, M.A., *Neuroscience: Exploring the Brain, 2nd edition*, Baltimore: Lippincott Williams and Wilkins, 2001

3. National Mental Health Association 2004 website.

4. The Cleveland Clinic website, 9500 Euclid Ave. NA31 Cleveland, OH 44195. 800-223-2273. 2004

8.5

STRESS BUSTERS

Always remember that striving and struggle precede success, even in the dictionary.

Sarah Ban Breathnach

As mentioned earlier, stress can have a serious impact on your health and well-being. As you read through the following suggestions remember that everyone is different. Some techniques may work for some and not for others. Also realize that reducing your stress will take some time and effort, everything worthwhile does. Some of these methods may produce immediate results but more than likely, reducing your stress will require incorporating certain stress reducing activities over time to see positive results.

Try to avoid stressful situations

If you have determined that certain situations cause you stress, try to eliminate them or change them if possible. For example, if you get worked up driving in heavy traffic talk to your boss and find out if you could come in 1 hour earlier and leave 1 hour earlier to avoid rush hour. If you have a newborn that is teething or colicky and won't stop crying and it is starting to produce stress, find out if a neighbor, family member, or friend can baby-sit for a few hours so you can "de-stress." If you find that paying bills at home is a stressful time, ask your partner/roommate/spouse to take over those duties for a while. The key here is to determine exactly what causes your stress. If you can change it or avoid it, do so.

Tackle one thing at a time

If you feel like you are being crushed under a mountain of things to do or are being pulled in too many directions at once, make a list of things you must do and finish each one before starting another. This will allow you to focus on each task at hand individually, instead of trying to do 50 things at once. This technique also creates a positive feeling. Checking off each of the things you have accomplished helps you to stay motivated.

Exercise

Exercise seems to be the modern cure-all for everything from weight loss to cardiac health, insomnia, and stress relief. Exercise is a cornerstone of the PRIME operating system for wellness but you may be surprised that only certain types of exercise lower stress, and only certain types of stress are best dealt with by exercise. According to Dr. Robert Goldman in his book *Brain Fitness,* moderate, low intensity exercise such as walking and tai-chi are much more effective at combating stress than high intensity workouts involving high heart rates, sweating, and straining.[1]

Moderate exercise is a more effective stress buster than high-intensity exercise because it doesn't set off stress hormones like cortisol and ACTH. It eases stress because it creates a mental "time-out" from the worries and pressures that cause stress. Moderate exercise may also act as a calming distraction, slowing the mind and body so that the entire system can stop its stressful churning.

But don't throw away your running shoes and barbells just yet. Any physical activity, intense, mild, or moderate is better than none. Numerous studies have shown that people who exercise regularly are more resistant to the effects of stress, and are able to bounce back from the effects of stress much more quickly than those who don't exercise. Intense or mild, regular exercise will delete the effects of stress and make you more resilient and able to cope with whatever life throws your way.

Take up a hobby

Take time for yourself by doing something that you enjoy. Try to make sure that it is low stress or a different kind of stress than what you are used to in order for your body to "re-set" its stress levels. Gardening, sewing, woodwork, lawn work, painting, dancing; even something competitive like tennis, golf, or bowling can help to take your mind off of your worries.

If you are unsure where to start, go to the hobby store. You may find something that interests you. Check with your local community center. They will often have classes for a small fee that can introduce you to a new hobby. Read the local paper for stories or ads from interesting groups that may be meeting in your area. Talk to your friends and ask what they do for fun, but beware, some people like their alone time. If they invite you to join them, then have fun. If they don't, try not to push them, and don't be offended. We each deal with stress in our own way.

Share your feelings

Research has shown that verbalizing your problems with another person, whether you are male or female can help you to de-stress, even if you don't find an answer to your problems. Simply talking with someone about how you feel can be like turning the knob on a pressure valve, letting go of some of the stress that was bothering you.

Talking to someone about your problems also helps you to define what you consider to be problems. Often times we may go through a period where we are upset by something and we don't even know what we are upset about. Something small may have set you off and after discussing it you may realize that that wasn't the problem at all. In addition, by verbally defining what is bothering you to someone else it may be easier to come up with a solution. After all, two heads are better than one.

In our age of hyper-independence, the "I can handle it myself" attitude may ultimately cause more stress than prevent it. Talk about your concerns, fears, and problems with someone you respect. You may find out that you are not the only one having a bad day. Allow your friends and family to help you and provide guidance, they may have solutions that you have not even thought of. I've found that friends and family are usually smarter than we think!

Be realistic

You can't accomplish everything no matter how hard you try. If you are feeling overwhelmed, learn to say no. You may be trying to take on more than you can or should handle. Tell your friends and family the reasons for saying "no" to some responsibilities and be ready to compromise on some activities. If you are meeting resistance to the changes you want to make, be flexible. You may need to rethink your position or strategy. If you think that you are correct, stand your ground, but do so calmly and rationally. If you are willing to give in, others may meet you halfway. Not only will you reduce stress, but you may find better solutions to your problems.[2]

Meditate

Tibetan monks consider meditation to be vital for their well-being, and they may be on to something. More and more research is piling up acknowledging the powerful affects of meditation. Anything that can lower your stress level is a useful tool but researchers are also finding significant physiological benefits as well. Meditation has been shown to lower your risk for heart disease, lower your stress levels, and improve your immune system function which enables you to fight off disease more effectively. Researchers at Harvard used MRI technology to examine the brain during meditation. What they found is that meditation often affects the part of your brain responsible for your autonomic nervous system, the part of your nervous system over which you seemingly have no control. Your autonomic nervous system controls such activities as digestion, heart rate, and blood pressure...all activities that can be negatively impacted by stress. Another research study found that meditation actually lowered the level of the stress hormone cortisol found in the blood stream after only 10 minutes of meditation.[3]

The major hurdle people have when initiating a meditation session is that they don't know if they are doing it right. The first thing to realize is that there really is no wrong way. If you feel better after doing it you are probably doing it right. The most common way to meditate is to sit quietly and concentrate on one thing such as your breathing while repeating a word, either aloud or to yourself. The word does not matter but some of the more popular words force you to expel a lot of air while saying them. Some examples are: Amen, One, or Om. Start slowly, begin by meditating for 5 minutes or so and gradually build yourself up to a comfortable amount of time. If you prefer to walk and meditate that is perfectly fine as well, simply find a quiet area where you can completely focus and not worry about any outside influences such as traffic or other people.

An important point about meditation or prayer—don't let it become a worry session. Often as we sit quietly our minds wander as we try to come up with solutions to our problems. Meditation is not the time for this, you are trying to de-stress yourself, not create more stress. Focus on your breathing while you are meditating and accept things the way they are. You have the other 23 hours in the day to worry.

Visualize

A powerful technique used by many successful people to combat stressful situations is to visualize yourself succeeding. For example, before a job interview prepare yourself by visualizing yourself in the interview on top of your game and ready to answer any question thrown at you. Picture everything going the way you want it to. At the same time, try to picture things not going exactly as planned. Prepare yourself for some unexpected scenarios. When they occur, and they most likely will, you will be that much more ready. This will help to calm you and lower the stress response happening in your body. While visualizing however, be sure not to focus on only the negative things that may happen as this can actually increase your stress level. Remain positive and confident about the situation and you will come out on top.

Another popular way to "de-stress" is to simply visualize yourself in a happy place. Picture yourself on a beach or watching a beautiful sunset. Concentrate on this image, slow your breathing, and relax your muscles. After just a few minutes you will feel the stress melt away.

Learn to relax, rest

As we talked about in a previous chapter, rest is crucial to YOU 1.0. So why can't we just relax? For many of us rest and relaxation just don't fit into our busy schedules. We have much more important things to do. When we do finally rest we may feel guilty about not doing some other things that need to be done. Many of us just aren't that good at relaxing. If that describes you, learn to relax. Set aside time each day that is *your* time. Don't let anything distract you from your relaxation time. Take a class about rest and relaxation at your local community center. Read a book about rest. Find a website, whatever, just learn to relax.

Learn to manage your time

Stress can be caused by any number of things. Big events such as a death in the family or a change of jobs are two common "big" events that cause a great deal of stress. More often than not however, everyday stress is the result of not having enough time and feeling rushed to get everything done. There are literally thousands of books, CD's, and products available that will help you to learn how to manage your time. What most of them have in common are three simple concepts: Prioritize, goal setting, learn to say no.

If you would like more information on the topic of time management two excellent books are *The Overwhelmed Person's Guide to Time Management* by Ronni Eisenberg and Kate Kelly, and *How to Get Control of Your Time and Your Life* by Alan Lakein. Both are easy reads with a tremendous amount of useful tips and information.

Cry

While humans intuitively have known for centuries that crying makes us feel better, a research study by William Frey, former Research Director of the St. Paul-Ramsey Dry Eye and Tear Research Center, was the first to scientifically confirm that people feel better after crying. 85% of females and 73% of males indicated that they feel better after shedding tears.

In crying episodes associated with sadness or anger, the subjects in the study reported an average reduction of emotional intensity of 40%. In other words, they felt 40% less sad or angry after crying. They also reported a reduction of intensity following crying episodes attributed to sympathy, anxiety, and fear. This is consistent with findings that people generally feel better after they cry. If emotional tearing reduces the effects of stress, then we may increase our susceptibility to a variety of physical and psychological problems when we suppress our tears.

One reason many older children and adults struggle so hard to control their tears is that they anticipate and often receive negative, non-supportive reactions from others. This lack of a positive reaction encourages the idea that crying indicates weakness, vulnerability, and immaturity.[4] This negative view on crying has gotten better as we have become a more sensitive society, but "tearing up" is still unfortunately looked down upon.

Crying can be a positive outlet for negative feelings. If you are unable to share your emotions with someone, find a quiet spot alone where you won't be disturbed and allow your feelings to express themselves freely. Don't hold back and go where your feelings take you. You will feel better afterwards.

Live a healthy lifestyle

As we have seen, stress can take its toll on you physically and mentally. By living a healthy lifestyle you can dramatically *decrease the affects of stress* as well as *lower your potential for stress*. Living a healthy lifestyle includes optimizing your Posture, Rest, Intake, Mind, and Exercise habits. When you focus on and utilize the PRIME operating system for YOU 1.0 you will feel and look better and you will be better prepared to handle any stressful situation that may occur.

Please note: Some of these techniques may sound too simplistic to be effective. That is not the case. Pick a few of the methods described above that you like to do, preferably techniques that you can practice throughout your lifetime. You will find that they are enjoyable as well as effective. As I tell many of my patients, just because it seems simple does not mean it is not effective. Just take a look at the wheel, or fruits and vegetables.

References

1. Goldman, Robert. *Brain Fitness.* DoubleDay, New York, 1999.

2. National Mental Health Association website 1-800-969-NMHA

3. Barbor, C. Psychology Today, May 2001.

4. http://www.e-well-being.com/index.html

9.0

IMPROVING MIND

Nothing can stop the man with the right mental attitude from achieving his goal; nothing on earth can help the man with the wrong mental attitude.

Thomas Jefferson

This chapter will focus on improving your awareness and appreciation for the things around you by improving your mind.

What could be more rewarding than improving your mind? Just like every other component of the PRIME operating system your mind can be improved and upgraded. Scientists have long known that as a child's brain is developing, it is creating new pathways and connections. Relatively new research shows that this is true of the adult brain as well. Connections between nerve cells that help us to recall memories, relate emotions, and react to different circumstances, are not "set in stone" or hardwired once they are created as we once thought. Neurons, or nerve cells, cannot reproduce themselves like other cells in your body, but they can grow stronger, bigger, and create different connections until the day we die. Our minds are constantly wiring, remodeling, and re-wiring as long as we are using them.

Researchers in Seattle and Boston who have been studying brain power and intellectual capacity for the last 45 years have proven that people who use their minds effectively and often, have the ability to think more quickly, remember more, and can grasp difficult concepts more easily than those who don't "exercise" their minds. Unlike a computer, you will never be stuck with an outdated or underpowered CPU. You can upgrade at any time with a little effort and knowledge. Just like any other organ or muscle in your body, the old saying "use it or lose it" applies to your brain. Almost any thing that is thought provoking or intellectually challenging can stimulate nerve growth and connectivity, which leads to increased mind power. The following tips and activities will encourage your brain to develop, and promote a healthy mind.

Read

Reading is not only a great way to relax, it also stimulates your mind. Whether you read educational material or purely for enjoyment, reading encourages the nerve cells in your brain to grow and form new connections with other brain cells. These new connections can help to create pathways for memories, emotions, and other intellectual functions controlled by your nervous system.

Reading helpful and insightful books (such as this one) can help you to increase your intelligence. Reading can also help you to unwind and relax, transporting you to a far away place or help you to solve a problem you've got. Use the knowledge of others to your advantage. Whether it is a self-help book or a fantasy, curl up with a good book tonight.

Education

Learning and education should be a lifelong project for everyone. Just because you have a diploma doesn't mean that you should stop learning. Take a class that interests you. If possible, go with your partner or a friend so that you will have something stimulating to talk about long after the class is over. Many colleges, community centers, and churches have courses you can take that cover nearly everything under the sun. Learn a foreign language and then take a trip to that country. Learn to knit or prepare your taxes. Educate yourself about human anatomy or nutrition. Learn how to sell your house yourself or how to wood-work. The opportunities are endless especially with the advent of the internet. What you decide to study is up to you, now get out there and learn something new today!

Live by the Golden Rule

What a wonderful world this would be if we all lived by the "Golden Rule."
Treat others as you would like to be treated.
When you treat others with dignity, compassion, and respect you will be rewarded with the same behavior directed towards you. Smile at others, pay attention to others when they are talking, be fair, and go the extra mile for someone else. You might be surprised at what you receive in return.

Laugh

Is laughter the best medicine? Not really, but it isn't too bad. Laughter and humor as medicine have received mixed reviews. There are those who believe that laughter can cure anything, and others who think that laughter as a remedy to any illness is wishful thinking. As research on this topic grows, there is one thing that most agree on, laughter sure can't hurt.

Studies have shown that hearty laughter increases your heart rate, breath rate, alertness, and exercises your skeletal muscles. After a period of laughter your heart rate, blood pressure, and muscle tone decreases resulting in increased relaxation. Humor can enhance your mood, sometimes for an extended period of time. Proponents of humor medicine also believe that laughing and humor can strengthen your immune system and reduce the amount of stress hormones being released and circulating within your body.[1] However it works, we all like to laugh, so do it more often.

Sunshine

Mankind has adapted to exposure to sunlight, and to a certain degree we are dependant on it for our health. We have become a society that spends more time indoors under artificial light than outdoors in the sun. As a result we may be setting ourselves up for a condition J. Ott described as "mal-illumination," a condition similar to malnutrition with similar health consequences.[2]

Sunlight, in small to moderate doses, has been linked to a multitude of healthy benefits. First, sunlight is the most important source for the formation of Vitamin D.[3] Vitamin D is formed in the subcutaneous fat layer underneath your skin when you are exposed to sunlight. Vitamin D is used by your body to help absorb calcium and phosphorus which are used to make and maintain strong bones and teeth. Research also suggests that vitamin D may help maintain a healthy immune system and help regulate cell growth and differentiation, the process that determines what a cell is to become.[4,5]

Second, small amounts of sunlight may help to keep your immune system working well. On the other hand, too much sunlight can harm your immune system making you more susceptible to infections as your body repairs the damage done by the UV rays.[6]

Finally, sunlight has been shown to raise the levels of serotonin in your brain and blood stream. Serotonin is a chemical your body produces which has been attributed to anti-depression.[7] Sunlight really can affect your mood and your mindset in a positive way.

If you want to enjoy the healthy benefits of sunlight please do so responsibly. Early morning and late evening are the best times to absorb sunlight because the rays are less intense and you are less susceptible to burning, a possible precursor to skin cancer. Ten to fifteen minutes of sunlight exposure allows adequate time for Vitamin D synthesis and should be followed by application of a sunscreen with an SPF of at least 15 to protect the skin. Ten to fifteen minutes of sun exposure at least two times per week to the face, arms, hands, or back, without sunscreen, is usually sufficient to provide adequate vitamin D.[8]

Change habits

Humans, like most animals, are creatures of habit. Break out of some of your routines for a while. If you take the same route to work every day or drop the kids off at school by taking the same path, mix it up. On your way, try to spot something you have never seen before. If you brush your teeth with one hand, use the other hand every now and again. If you typically exercise before work, try to workout after work or during lunch. Use the other ear for phone conversations. Practice writing your name with your non-dominant hand. Read a book upside down. While waiting for your gas tank to fill up stand on one foot. Eat lunch with your left hand only. Have fun and mix things up a little, you only live once.

Increase physical exercise

An interesting study performed at the Duke University Medical Center found that brisk exercise for 30 minutes three times a week was as effective as, or more effective than Zoloft® for treating depression. The researchers followed 156 older patients who had been diagnosed with major depression. After 16 weeks, much to the researchers' surprise, they found that the patients who exercised showed statistically significant improvement compared to those who took anti-depression medication and those who took the medication and combined it with exercise.[9] Exercise not only benefits you physically but mentally as well.

The following are some additional ways to keep your mind running at optimum capacity for many years to come.

- Balance your checkbook by hand
- Learn a musical instrument
- Keep lists
- Volunteer for a cause you believe in
- Add one word of vocabulary per week
- Stay informed about what's going on in the world
- Memorize a song or poem
- Enjoy simple things like playing games with others or a sunset
- Do something for another
- Learn to listen when interacting with people
- Switch careers or start a new one
- Learn a foreign language

References

1. Goldman, Robert, *Brain Fitness.* Double Day, New York, 1999.

2. McGhee, Paul. *Health, Healing and the Amuse System: Humor as Survival Training*, Kendall/Hunt Dubuque, IA 1999.

3. Ott, JN. *Light, Radiation and You: How to Stay Healthy.* Devin-Adair Publishers, Greenwich, CT, 1990.

4. Holick MF. McCollum Award Lecture, 1994: *Vitamin D: new horizons for the 21st century.* Am J Clin Nutr 1994;60:619-30.

5. Holick MF. *Evolution and function of vitamin D. Recent Results* Cancer Res 2003;164:3-28.

6. Hayes CE, Hashold FE, Spach KM, Pederson LB. *The immunological functions of the vitamin D endocrine system.* Cell Mol Biol 2003;49:277-300.

7. Lambert GW, Reid C, Kaye DM, Jennings GL, Esler MD. *Effect of sunlight and season on serotonin turnover in the brain.* Lancet. 2002 Dec 7;360(9348):1840-2.

8. Holick MF. *Vitamin D: the underappreciated D-lightful hormone that is important for skeletal and cellular health.* Curr Opin Endocrinol Diabetes 2002;9:87-98.

9. Michael Babyak, James A. Blumenthal, Steve Herman, Parinda Khatri, Murali Doraiswamy, Kathleen Moore, W. Edward Craighead, Teri T. Baldewicz, and K. Ranga Krishnan. *Exercise Treatment for Major Depression: Maintenance of Therapeutic Benefit at 10 Months.* Psychosomatic Medicine, September/October 2000.

10.0

EXERCISE

Those who do not find time for exercise will have to find time for illness.

Earl of Derby

Exercise is the final component of the PRIME operating system for YOU 1.0 and is as important as the other four components: Posture, Rest, Intake, and Mental well-being. In fact, exercise may be the one universal truth that researchers, scientists, doctors, nutritionists, psychiatrists, and all other disciplines related to heath care can agree on. Physical activity was ranked at the top of the list of the top 10 leading health indicators by *Healthy People 2010*, a health initiative sponsored by the Presidents Council on Physical Fitness and the Centers for Disease Control. (The complete list is located to the right.) Physical activity, in addition to being listed in the top ten health indicators, also has an effect on other indicators such as obesity and mental health, making it that much more important.

Exercise, if done safely and correctly, is good for you. It can help to make you stronger, less susceptible to disease and injury, alter your mood, and basically help you to live a healthier and longer life. In this chapter we will focus on just what exactly exercise is, why it is good for us, and the different components that make up physical fitness.

U.S. Healthy People 2010 Ten Leading Health Indicators
1. Physical Activity
2. Overweight & Obesity
3. Tobacco
4. Substance Abuse
5. Responsible Sexual Behavior
6. Mental Health
7. Injury and Violence
8. Environmental Quality
9. Immunization
10. Access to Health Care

Healthy People 2010, Physical Activity and Fitness. *PCPFS Research Digest*. Series 3, No. 13. March 2001.

Exercise can come in many different forms and has many different definitions. Generally, physical exercise is considered to be any activity that requires physical exertion when performed to develop or maintain fitness. Just thinking about exercise makes some people cringe. We know it is good for us, and yet we just can't seem to establish a regular pattern of exercise. Over 50% of Americans don't exercise at a level that is beneficial to their health and 30% of Americans don't exercise at all according to the National Centers for Disease Control and Prevention.[1] It has been reported that as many as 250,000 lives are lost per year because of a sedentary lifestyle. That is more than the number of lives lost due to accidents, influenza, and pneumonia combined.[2]

Technology has certainly made our lives easier, but it has also decreased our level of physical fitness. We lead more sedentary lives that require less physical activity than previous generations. Our parents and grandparents probably stayed relatively fit through their daily work routine. Today, most of us sit at a desk all day staring into a computer screen, hardly a rigorous workout. Getting and staying in shape doesn't require a gym membership or fancy equipment, but it does require effort. Later we will discuss why we don't exercise and some tips to help overcome those reasons. For now, let's examine what exercise does so that we can better understand why it is so vital to YOU 1.0.

Exercise requires physical exertion which in turn requires your muscles to perform work. When your muscles work you are burning calories, in essence, expending energy. Your body uses energy derived from food and energy storage in 3 different ways.

1. The first way you expend energy is through your basal metabolic rate. Your basal metabolic rate represents the energy required to carry out your normal bodily functions such as breathing, keeping your heart beating, and maintaining muscular tone. For sedentary individuals this is where the majority of energy is expended, roughly 50-70% of daily energy expenditure.

2. The second way we burn calories or expend energy is through the thermic effect of food. When we digest and absorb the food we have eaten, our baseline temperature goes up, producing heat and expending energy. The thermic effect of food only accounts for 5-10% of our total energy expenditure over a 24 hour period.

3. The final way we expend energy, and the only one which we have control over, is through physical activity. The amount of energy expended by physical activity during a 24 hour period depends on the duration and intensity of the exercise. Simply put, the more your muscles work, the more energy you will burn. In a sedentary person approximately 30% of our daily energy expenditure goes towards physical activity. If you are much more active and engage in regular exercise and physical activity you can increase your energy expenditure by 100% or more.[3]

So what is actually happening to our bodies when we exercise and why does it take so much energy? Remember back when we discussed metabolism as the total amount of chemical reactions taking place in every cell in our body? Exercise, simply put, requires more chemical reactions to take place to supply all of our cells with the ingredients necessary to sustain themselves and perform the tasks that are required of them. Increasing the number of chemical reactions requires more oxygen, breakdown of energy storage reserves, and an increased blood flow to distribute all of the ingredients to the right places. To illustrate the degree to which our metabolism increases through exercise think of this: In an individual with an extremely high fever the body metabolism increases about 100% above normal. By comparison, the metabolism of the body during a marathon race increases to 2000% percent above normal![4]

In addition to increasing your metabolism, exercise also increases the strength of tissues in your body, most notably your muscles and bones, (remember that your heart is a muscle.) Unless you exercise on a regular basis, you begin to lose muscle mass after the age of 30. After 30, you will lose approximately 3-5% of your muscle mass every 10 years. Bones benefit from weight bearing exercise as well. Bone mass increases with increased amounts of exercise which can help to fight osteoporosis and osteomalacia. Bone mass reaches maximum density between the ages of 25-40. After the age of 40 bone mass declines at about ½% per year. Remember the old saying use it or lose it? Our bodies are in a constant state of replacement and renewal. If you don't use it you will lose it. Our inborn intelligence is so smart that our bodies monitor the use of certain tissues and anticipate and forecast usage in the future to conserve energy and nutrients. Think about it like this: You are the manager of operations for all of the resources in your body. It is your responsibility to make sure that all systems have the materials they need. Not any extra because that would be inefficient, and not too little or that could result in system failure and decreased productivity. Given this scenario, if you don't exercise or perform weight bearing activity it would be silly to keep sending orders and supplies to maintain and build new muscle and bone once you have finished growing. If you are active however, you must maintain your muscle and bone structure to keep up with the demands put on them.

Exercise and your heart

Heart disease or coronary artery disease is a major cause of death in the United States. In fact, one out of two Americans dies from a cardiovascular disease.[5] Cardiovascular disease is not necessarily a disease of the elderly as some may think. It is the leading cause of death in men between the ages of 35 and 44, and the incidence of cardiovascular disease in women has risen dramatically in the last few years. To put it in perspective Cardiovascular disease (CVD) killed 945,836 Americans in 2000. Other major causes of death in 2000 were: cancer, 553,091; accidents, 97,900; Alzheimer's disease, 49,558; and HIV (AIDS) 14,478. In the case of women, 1 in 29 women's deaths is from breast cancer, while 1 in 2.4 is from CVD.

What is Cardiovascular disease?

There are virtually hundreds of types of cardiovascular diseases but the majority of disabilities and deaths are the result of four of the most common: Atherosclerosis, Coronary Heart disease, Hypertension, and Stroke. It is not the scope of this book to go into great detail about each one of these diseases but a short discussion may be helpful.

- Atherosclerosis is not a single disease but a group of diseases characterized by plaque build-up, hardening, and narrowing of arteries, the blood vessels that carry oxygen and nutrient rich blood to all parts of your body. Atherosclerosis comes from the Greek words *athero* meaning gruel or paste, and *sclerosis* meaning hardness.[6] Atherosclerosis is a progressive disease where cholesterol, calcium, fatty deposits, and cell debris collect on the vessel wall causing a restriction of blood flow. The dangers of atherosclerosis are when the vessel becomes blocked depriving an area of vital supplies, or when the plaque ruptures and creates a clot which can break off and flow into a smaller vessel causing blockage there. The development of severe atherosclerosis in the arteries supplying blood to the heart is the cause of almost all heart attacks. Widespread atherosclerosis throughout your arteriole supply system also causes your heart to work harder as signals are sent from areas that are not getting the oxygen and nutrients that they need, forcing your heart to pump harder and faster.

- Coronary Heart disease is a form of atherosclerosis that affects a specific set of arteries, namely the coronary arteries that supply blood to your heart. Severe blockage of coronary arteries can lead to the formation of a blood clot which can completely block the artery leading to a myocardial infarction or heart attack. A heart attack is the destruction and death of heart muscle cells because they didn't receive the nutrients they constantly require.

- Hypertension is the medical term for high blood pressure. High blood pressure causes the heart to work harder than normal to pump blood to tissues and organs. When this happens the heart and arteries are more susceptible to injury. High blood pressure can also cause the heart to grow bigger and less efficient. High blood pressure damages arteries caus-

Risk factors for cardiovascular disease
The good news is that many of the risk factors for CVD can be modified and treated. Remember, the more risk factors you have the higher your chances for developing some type of CVD.
• Physical inactivity
• Smoking
• High blood cholesterol
• Obesity/overweight
• Diabetes
• Male gender
• Increasing age
• Stress response
• Heredity
• Excessive alcohol
• Certain drugs (legal and illegal)
• Menopause

ing scarring and hardening which limits blood flow to the tissues in your body.

♦ A stroke is a cardiovascular disease that affects the brain. A stroke occurs when a blood vessel supplying the brain becomes clogged by a blood clot or when a vessel becomes weakened and ruptures. This blockage or rupture deprives the delicate nerve cells in your brain of oxygen and nutrients which can result in nerve cell death within minutes. Strokes can be especially devastating because nerve cells don't grow back once they die.

The effects of exercise on the cardiovascular system

♥ Contrary to popular belief, moderate exercise does not directly affect the heart as much as you might think. Of course there are direct benefits, such as an increase in heart efficiency and an increase in the number of collateral or "helper" coronary arteries supplying the heart with blood. But, many of the major benefits of exercise on your cardiovascular system are found elsewhere in your body.

♥ Exercise helps to increase your lung volume and blood cell volume. This increased lung and blood cell volume decreases the amount of work your heart has to do to deliver oxygen to the tissues of your body.

♥ Exercise may also increase the size and elasticity of blood vessels which can help to lower blood pressure and decrease the work load of your heart. Many people think of their blood vessels as little copper pipes that carry blood throughout the body. This is not quite the case. Blood vessels are actually quite dynamic. They are constantly changing shape and size to accommodate the demands placed on the various tissues of the body. They expand and contract, and some blood vessels even have valves in them to regulate distribution. Atherosclerosis limits the ability of the blood vessels to change size and affects how hard your heart must pump to deliver blood.

♥ Regular physical activity burns calories which helps you to lose excess body fat. As body fat is lost and lean muscle mass is added, your body is better equipped to metabolize the fat you intake. The increased ability to use the fat you intake for energy instead of storing it for later use decreases your risk of developing atherosclerosis.

* Remember, these benefits are linked to regular physical activity, not random acts of activity.

Fast facts, Your Heart

Your heart is the most powerful muscle in your body. As you exercise, your body needs more blood which delivers vital nutrients, increasing your heart rate. While you are exercising and strengthening your heart think of these facts:

♥ The human heart beats about 40 million times per year.

♥ By the time you reach 70 your heart will have beat 2.8 billion times-all without taking a break!

♥ Your heart pumps about 1 million barrels, or over 48 million gallons of blood during your lifetime. That is enough to fill more than 3 supertankers. Not bad for a pump that lasts 80+ years and weighs about 10 ounces!

Exercise as a stress release

One of the most effective ways to combat stress is through exercise. Exercise, especially aerobic exercise which increases your heart and breath rate, has also been shown to relieve mild depression and helps people to cope during difficult times. Clinicians have seen that one exercise session can generate 90-120 minutes of relaxation response due to the release of endorphins and certain neurotransmitters. What that means is that the electrical activity in your muscles decreases after exercise, leaving you less jittery and hyperactive while at the same time your mood improves and you are able to relax.

Aren't up for aerobic exercise? Don't worry, activities such as yoga can have stress-busting capabilities as well. Typically, during yoga and yoga like activities you gradually increase the work your muscles are doing while gradually relaxing your mind. Studies have shown that when large muscle groups repeatedly contract and relax, the brain receives a signal to release specific neurotransmitters, which in turn make you feel more relaxed and alert.

Exercise and Stress—Added Benefit: Scientists know that stress causes the release of certain hormones which cause you to release glucose (your body's main energy sugar) into your blood stream. If the glucose is not used up immediately your body responds by secreting insulin telling your body to store the excess energy in the form of fat. Exercise helps to not only burn excess calories but to inhibit the stress response which actually can promote weight gain.[7]

If you are looking to exercise to help you reduce stress remember this: exercise can also <u>be</u> stressful! To help you cope with stress try to pick an exercise that doesn't cause stress. For example, if you don't really like crowds, don't think that you have to join a busy gym. Pick something fun that you like to do and exercise solo. If you stress out about making it to a class on time choose an activity that you can do in your spare time at home. Exercise is for *you*, make it about you and not everyone else.

Exercise, Diabetes & Obesity

According to the FDA, at least 10 million people in the U.S. at high risk for developing Type II diabetes can sharply lower their chances for getting this disease through exercise and improved dietary habits. Type II diabetes, also known as Adult Onset Diabetes, is thought to be caused by an increased resistance to insulin as we gain weight. This increased resistance to insulin makes it harder for our bodies to regulate our blood sugar. Adult onset diabetes accounts for 90-95 percent of all diabetes cases in the United States. It occurs mostly in middle/older age adults and in people who are overweight. A majority of people who are overweight have some degree of insulin resistance, but only a portion develop diabetes.

Exercise has been shown to increase your body's ability to use insulin as much as twofold. How this happens is not exactly understood. Exercise also aids weight reduction, a further benefit in controlling diabetes.

Exercise and Cancer

Exercise and cancer, two of the most frightening words in the English language. Everyone wants to know how to lower their risk for developing cancer. Researchers have only recently begun to understand the benefits of exercise relating to the decreased risk of being diagnosed with some type of cancer. In the case of breast cancer, the second leading cause of cancer related death in women just behind lung cancer, exercise may lower the risk significantly. This is thought to occur on two levels. First, extra fat makes extra estrogen which can actually promote the growth of some breast cancers. Regular exercise can help to maintain weight gain so you don't have the extra estrogen producing fat. Second, researchers have found that regular exercise can help to regulate circulating estrogen levels, in some cases lowering it to more acceptable levels.

Further research on exercise and cancer has found that exercise helps to boost your immune system which is responsible for weeding out abnormal cells and toxins. For those diagnosed with cancer, exercise can help to prevent weight gain or loss from chemotherapy and help with treatment side effects.

Exercise, flexibility and endurance

Exercise also increases your flexibility. As we age the elasticity of our muscles, tendons, and ligaments decreases. Think of a sponge as it dries out. It becomes stiff, hard, and less flexible. The same concept applies to your muscles and your joints. Proper exercise and stretching helps to lubricate joints and keep muscles from getting tight and achy. Exercise and stretching can also decrease you risk of injury, increase your range of motion, and decrease joint pain.

Another benefit to regular physical activity is increased endurance. Endurance is the ability to perform a task for an extended period of time without experiencing fatigue. For some, the goal of physical endurance may be to run a marathon. For others it may be to climb a flight of stairs without getting winded. Whatever your goals, exercise can slow or even prevent the eventual decline of your physical endurance.

Add it up...
Healthy Lifestyle + Exercise = Longevity and increased quality of life

Perhaps the most significant reason to exercise and stay physically fit is because it seems to be a major factor in prolonging life, AND increasing the quality of life by decreasing the risk of heart disease, diabetes, cancer, osteoporosis, and countless other diseases we are faced with every day. Regular physical activity can improve your state of mind, self confidence, physical independence, and decrease depression.

The primary benefit of exercise is that it is <u>FOR YOU 1.0</u>. It helps YOU 1.0 to look good and it makes YOU 1.0 feel good.

Exercise does guarantee good health

References

1. CA Macera, PhD, DA Jones, PhD, MM Yore, MSPH, SA Ham, MS, HW Kohl, PhD, CD Kimsey, Jr, PhD, D Buchner, MD, Div of Nutrition and Physical Activity, National Center for Chronic Disease Prevention and Health Promotion, CDC. *Prevalence of Physical Activity, Including Lifestyle Activities Among Adults* United States, 2000—2001 MMWR August 15, 2003, 52(32):764–769.

2. U.S. Centers for Disease Control National Center for Health Statistics, 2001.

3. Champe, PC, Harvey, RA, *Biochemistry 2nd Ed.* Lippincott-Raven, Philadelphia, 1994.

4. Guyton & Hall, *Textbook of Medical Physiology 9th ed.* W.B.Saunders Co. Philadelphia, 1996.

5. American Heart Association. *Heart Disease and Stroke Statistics—2004 Update.* Dallas, Tex.: American Heart Association; 2003.

6. *Heart and Stroke Facts*, American Heart Association, page 3, 2003.

7. Facchini FS, et al. *Hyperinsulinemia: the missing link among oxidative stress and age-related diseases?* Free Radic Biol Med 2000 Dec;29(12):1302-6.

11.0

IMPROVING EXERCISE

If we could give every individual the right amount of nourishment and exercise, not too little and not too much, we would have found the safest way to health.

Hippocrates

Before engaging in any exercise program you should consult your physician.

O.K., you have decided that exercise may actually be good for you and you would like to make it a part of your healthy lifestyle. But…you're not sure what to do and where to start. In this chapter we will discuss how to start an exercise program right for you, which exercises will suit your needs, how to stay motivated, and some common excuses you will eventually come up with for not exercising.

Before starting an exercise program, or even if you exercise currently, it is important to have goals in mind. They don't have to be specific goals such as: I want to be able to climb Mt. Everest in 3 weeks, or I want to be able to bench press 400 pounds by December. Just having some goal in mind will help you to stay focused. Simply saying "I want to be healthier" may work for some people but for many it is too broad of a concept to grasp and too hard to measure concretely. Instead, make getting healthier your general goal, and to do that set measurable goals that you can see, feel, and touch. Some examples may be:

- To fit into your wedding, prom, cocktail, dress again
- Be able to jog five miles without stopping
- Lose 10 pounds
- Lower your blood pressure by 10 points
- Touch your toes without pain
- Eliminate back pain
- Compete in a fun run for charity with your friends

Where do I start?

If you haven't exercised for a long time, or ever, are overweight, and have a high risk of some type of chronic health problem, see your doctor for a medical evaluation before beginning a physical activity program. Once you have determined that it is O.K. to exercise pick an activity that you enjoy. A sample list of some activities is provided below to get you thinking. The best exercise is one that you can and will do regularly, and one you enjoy doing. The list below is not exhaustive by any means. Almost any activity that gets your heart beating, makes you breathe a little harder, and causes you to sweat a little can be good exercise. The way you exercise is only limited by your imagination.

Swimming	Racquetball	Tennis	Walking
Jogging	Cycling	Basketball	Skiing
Dancing	Gardening	Ping Pong	Aerobics
Tai Chi'	Sit-ups	Weight lifting	Volleyball
Horseshoes	Stretching	Golf	Kickboxing
Jump rope	Soccer	Hiking	Yard work
Play Frisbee	Jumping Jacks	Skating	Aqua Aerobics
Housework	Gymnastics	Play Catch	Swinging
Baseball	Sledding	Yoga	Hopscotch
Boxing	Ballet	Karate	Badminton

What kind of exercise is best for me and my goals?

Goals, that darn buzzword that is so hard for many of us to grasp. We think that we know how to set goals, and we might. The hard part comes from trying to reach those goals. If our goals are too lofty we will get discouraged and give up. If they are set too low we lose interest because the challenge is gone.

To set physical activity goals, start exercising and stick with it for at least one week. Just have fun and enjoy yourself. Then, after you have determined an activity that you enjoy and have gotten a baseline of where you stand currently, set your goals. This will help you to set more appropriate goals.

Some common goals might be:

+ Run without stopping in an upcoming charity event.
+ Become more healthy (A great goal, but somewhat abstract. That is why it is important to find out where you are at now so you will notice as improvements are made.)
+ Lose 5/10/15 pounds.
+ Exercise 3 times per week.

> **Download NOW:**
> Write your goals down and put them in a place that you will see everyday. This will help to remind you and motivate you. Remember, just because they are written down doesn't mean that they can't be modified to meet changing situations.

Whatever your goals are make sure that they are realistic and realize that they are not set in stone. They can be modified to meet changing situations and circumstances. Also realize that when you begin to exercise you will make mistakes and slip-ups. You will skip a few workouts, you may lose motivation, and you may lose some fitness ground that you had gained. This is normal. Don't get discouraged and give up. Get back on track and start making progress again as soon as you can.

Now that your goals are set you will probably have a strong idea of what kind of exercise to partake in. If your goals are not exercise or sport dependent (like "I want to run in a 10K), you should determine what kind of physical activity will be most beneficial for you.

If you want to exercise for purely health benefits nearly any activity will do. Research has shown that even low levels of physical activity will have a positive impact on your health. If you are exercising to lose weight, an activity that is a little more vigorous and longer lasting (+30 minutes per session) will help to burn calories quicker and increase your metabolism.

> **Fast Fact:**
> It takes about 3500 calories burned to lose one pound of fat.

Walking, elliptical training, bicycling, and swimming are excellent examples. If you are having trouble determining what type of exercise to partake in, talk to a physical trainer or your physician for help.

I don't want too…12.5 common excuses and ways to motivate yourself

I just don't feel like it. I'll do it later. I don't have enough time. Most of us can rationalize why we don't want to exercise or give a reason why we can't. Listen, we all have things to do in our lives, what it boils down to is the level of priority you put on your daily activities. Think of the things you enjoy doing today. Picking the kids up from school, completing a tough assignment for your boss, spending quality time with your loved ones, or simply playing with your dog. Now imagine if your health didn't allow you to do these activities because you didn't take steps to enhance it. Regret is something we feel when it is too late. Don't regret tomorrow that you didn't keep yourself in shape today. Below you will find the top 12.5 reasons why people don't exercise and some tips on how to break through those excuses.

1. You don't have enough time.

With all of our so-called time saving devices it is a wonder that we don't have more than enough time to fit in a little physical activity. Unless your day is jam packed with things for you to do (watching TV and talking on the phone don't count), you have time to exercise, you simply need to find it. Walk and talk while you are on the phone, you can walk around the house or around the block while you are talking to aunt Jenny for a half hour. If you have to take care of the kids, involve them. Take them to a gym that has a daycare and activities for them, or let them help you count your reps. You may be surprised at how active they become helping you to stay motivated. And remember, you don't have to exercise all at once. Break up your workouts into 2–15 minute sessions or 3–10 minute sessions.

2. You are too embarrassed

Forget that you can't run as far as the next girl. Ignore the fact that you can't lift as much weight as that guy. No one cares how you look in your workout clothes as much as you do. Keep in mind, you are exercising for yourself. If you can't bring yourself to put on that spandex outfit in the gym locker room, find a private option you might enjoy. Rent or buy some inexpensive videos or some equipment to use at home. Walk or jog around your block. If you are self-conscious about your neighbors seeing you, bike or drive to another neighborhood. They won't mind.

3. You find exercise boring

Doing the same thing over and over, whether it is at work or in your exercise routine, can get repetitive. Don't make exercise a chore, something you have to do rather than something you want to do. Have fun, and instead of picking one physical activity you enjoy, pick two or three and alternate between them. Or, find a buddy you can chat with while you work out. Watch your favorite television program while you workout. Download new music to listen to. Even a dog can help to break up the routine. Pick a comfortable walking route around your neighborhood. When your dog "makes" pick it up (you do clean up after him/her don't you?) and jog the rest of the way home. If you're like me, you want to get rid of it as soon as you can.

4. You have health problems

Talk to your doctor. Regular physical activity can actually help many health conditions such as asthma, obesity, high blood pressure, and diabetes. Talk to your physician before starting any exercise program. Unless there is a specific reason for you not too exercise at some level, your doctor will probably be all for it.

5. You are always too tired

This problem itself may stem from lack of exercise. Physical inactivity can cause feelings of fatigue and tiredness. A regular program of exercise can help to boost your metabolism giving you more energy. If possible, try to exercise in the morning when you are more refreshed instead of at the end of a long day.

6. You feel that you get enough exercise already

Examine what you do at home and at work already. If you raise your heart level into your target zone for 20 minutes at a time 3-5 times a week you may indeed get enough exercise. If you don't, then no excuse for you.

7. You don't like to exercise because it hurts

Exercise, if done properly shouldn't hurt. You may experience stiffness and soreness if you haven't exercised in a while a day or two after exercising, this is very normal. If you have experienced pain while exercising talk to your doctor. You may simply need to slow down a bit. Keep in mind that you don't have to go 100% to receive the benefits of physical activity. Exercise doesn't have to be grueling. You should be able to carry on a conversation without losing your breath if you are exercising at a moderate level.

8. You just don't feel like it

There are days when you just say, "Ahh, I'll do it tomorrow, I don't feel like it today." When you reach that point it is important to remember why you are exercising. That may help to motivate you. If that doesn't work, use rewards to keep you on track. Going out to dinner on Saturday night after a successful week of exercise or going to a movie can be good rewards for some people. You may be able to make a deal with your spouse to watch the kids while you go shopping for a fun new outfit or out with your friends if you complete your exercise program. How about a massage? That new CD you've been wanting? A weekend getaway? Get creative with your rewards program and make a deal with your spouse, a friend, or yourself. Remember, you aren't a dog, a reward doesn't necessarily mean food.

Another way to motivate yourself is to use the buddy system. Work out with a friend. That way you have to answer to someone other than yourself at the end of the day. The feelings of not wanting to let a friend down can be a powerful motivator for both of you.

9. You are too old

First of all you are never too old to exercise. You may not be able to lift 100 pounds over your head or sprint down the block like you once could, but there are many different things you can do. Unfortunately, humans can be pretty stubborn creatures. Don't stop exercising because you can't do what you used to. Accept the fact that you are aging and find a new activity. Water aerobics, walking, tai chi', and stretching are all good low impact/low stress exercises if your body doesn't quite perform like it used to.

Second, exercise is beneficial at any age. It has been shown to increase longevity and quality of life in people of all ages. It may also boost your energy levels, help you to lose weight and take some stress off of your joints. Exercise can even be a positive influence on your mental health. Find something you can do safely and something you enjoy doing. Exercise is not age specific.

> We all want things quickly and with as little effort as possible. Be glad that your body doesn't work that way though because we would have to take the bad with the good. I for one am happy that every time I eat a Krispy Kreme doughnut I don't immediately go up a waist size. Enjoy your doughnut or your "no-no" food every once in awhile and thank your body for working the way it does.

10. You aren't seeing any changes

Becoming healthy, gaining muscle mass, and losing weight takes time. You didn't suddenly wake up with an extra 10 pounds around your mid-section did you? My gosh I hope not! In our society of instant gratification we want results NOW. Our bodies don't work that way. Believe me, I wish I could walk into a gym, work out, and walk out the door physically fit. It will take time to see and feel the changes that are taking place within your body. Embrace that fact and accept it because there are no quick fixes or short cuts.

11. You think that exercise is a waste of time

Think of exercise as regular maintenance for your health. It is astounding to me that Americans will spend approximately $2000 per year on car maintenance. $2000 per year on a hunk of metal and plastic that they will keep for about 4-6 years. Yet, some of these same people will spend next to nothing and no time on themselves, the only body they will have for their entire life. Make a vow to yourself that the next time you get the oil changed in your car you are going to start a regular maintenance program for yourself.

If you think that you have too much to do or that exercise is wasting valuable time that you could spend doing something else, try multi-tasking. Talk on the phone while you are on the treadmill. Write out the grocery list while you are on your stationary bike. Go over that important presentation in your head as you jog. Read a book or a report while on the Stairmaster. Do lunges in your office while you are waiting for your computer to reboot. Bring 10 pound weights to the office and do curls while talking on speaker phone. Again, get creative. When you are doing something for your health and well being it is never a waste of time. Do something, do anything.

12. You can't afford a gym membership

By now you should have realized that you don't need to go to a gym or class, or participate in a formal exercise program to realize the benefits of regular physical activity. With little to no monetary investment you can be up and running, literally. Buy a good pair of shoes for the activity you will be doing and you should be all set. Of course you can spend an unlimited amount on equipment, memberships, trainers and the like but you don't have to. Just do what you have to do to get moving.

12.5 You don't know how to exercise

Sorry, that excuse doesn't cut it. You have a wealth of information available today, virtually at your fingertips. Rent a video, read a book, or use the internet to research a safe activity that appeals to you. You are limited only by your imagination.

Download Now…
10.6 Easy Ways to Fit Exercise into Your Busy Schedule

1. Take the stairs instead of the elevator and climb a little faster than you might normally. Remember, folks used to actually HAVE to use the stairs before elevators and escalators. Now it seems the only time we use them is when we are on a Stairmaster and we aren't actually going anywhere. To "step" it up a notch, take the stairs two at a time. That will really get your heart pumping.
2. Count your steps. Buy a pedometer and try to work your way up to 10,000 steps during the day. (About 5 miles). Counting your steps will keep you motivated to try and "beat" your previous record.
3. Walk your dog. If you don't have a dog, consider getting one or offer to walk the neighbor's dog. They are tireless motivators and once their routine is established they will pester you until you take them for a walk. Trust me, my dog Scout lets me know when we haven't taken our daily walk.
4. Park at the back of the lot. You might be surprised at how many steps you and your kids take by parking a little ways away from where you are headed. Instead of driving around for 5 minutes looking for the perfect spot, park a little ways away and walk. While you're at it, skip the pay at the pump at the gas station, the drive-thru at the bank and the pharmacy, and get out of your car to run your errands. Who knows, you might run into an old friend who owes you some money. (By the way, tell them about this great book you just read.☺)
5. Use a cordless or cell phone and walk around while talking at home or at the office. While pacing around the house for 15-20 minutes talking to Aunt Jenny you could cover over a mile in distance and burn almost 100 calories.
6. When sitting or standing for a long period of time, practice pushing or pulling against immovable objects like a wall or a desk bolted down. This is called isometric exercise when your muscles contract fully without actually moving. You can isometrically contract your abs, glutes (rear end), and almost any major muscle group as you sit at your desk, on the couch, or even in the car. This can be great for muscle toning but just make sure that if you are using an object for resistance it really is *immovable*, we don't want you knocking down a wall now do we Hercules?
7. Consider TV time activity time. When it's on, do something. Stretch, do sit-ups during the commercials, jump rope, or move that old stationary

bike out of the garage and ride it while you watch. You can do almost any activity you can think of while you watch TV.

8. Take a walk for 20-30 minutes during your lunch hour, preferably before you eat. You will burn some calories and increase your metabolism before you consume your meal helping to stabilize your blood sugar and increase the rate at which you burn calories.

9. Turn your household chores into fun exercise time. Turn on some music and "Get Down" as you vacuum, clean the windows, and fold the laundry. Wash your car by hand instead of driving through the car wash. Mow the lawn yourself, or better yet, buy a cheap manual mower. If you let your grass go for a couple of weeks you are talking serious workout! Scrub the shower and really put your back and arms into it. By combining your chores with exercise you will have more fun doing both, and you will probably finish them more quickly.

10. Use a basket or a re-usable bag when shopping instead of a shopping cart. First of all you won't be able to fit as much junk food in there, and second you will tone your muscles as you shop.

10.5 If you have finished your isometric exercises at your desk or sitting at home try this, sit on the edge of your seat, couch, whatever, and extend one leg straight out. With your big toe trace the alphabet. Do this slowly and deliberately in big letters. When you are finished with one leg switch to the other leg.

10.6 This book weighs about ½ pound. Not a whole heck of a lot, but a nice weight to carry around with you swinging your arms as you walk around the block. Don't forget to show all of your friends and neighbors what you are carrying.

This list is certainly not exhaustive, although if you do all of these tips you may become exhausted. Get a little creative and I'm sure you can think of many more ways to fit in fitness.

Below is a chart that you can use to calculate how many calories you will burn performing an activity you enjoy.

Energy Expenditure Chart
1. Sedentary Activities Energy Costs

1. Sedentary Activities	Energy Costs Cals/Hour*
Lying down or sleeping	90
Sitting quietly	84
Sitting and writing, card playing, etc.	114
2. Moderate Activities	(150-350)
Bicycling (5 mph)	174
Canoeing (2.5 mph)	174
Dancing (Ballroom)	210
Golf (2-some, carrying clubs)	324
Horseback riding (sitting to trot)	246
Light housework, cleaning, etc.	246

Swimming (crawl, 20 yards/min)	288
Tennis (recreational doubles)	312
Volleyball (recreational)	264
Walking (2 mph)	198
3. Vigorous Activities	**More than 350**
Aerobic Dancing	546
Basketball (recreational)	450
Bicycling (13 mph)	612
Circuit weight training	756
Football (touch, vigorous)	498
Ice Skating (9 mph)	384
Racquetball	588
Roller Skating (9 mph)	384
Jogging (10 minute mile, 6 mph)	654
Scrubbing Floors	440

Swimming (crawl, 45 yards/min)	522
Tennis (recreational singles)	450
X-country Skiing (5 mph)	690

*Hourly estimates based on values calculated for calories burned per minute for a 150 pound (68 kg) person.

To find the number of calories you would burn up in any of the activities noted on the previous chart: Take your weight and divide by 150. Multiply this number by the number of calories burned in an hour of an activity you like to do that is listed on the chart. This will give you the number of calories YOU 1.0 burn doing this activity for an hour.

Your weight/150 = x times calories burned = # of calories you will burn.

For example if you weigh 136 pounds and you played doubles tennis for 1 hour you would burn 282 calories. 136/150=.91 x 312 = 282 calories per hour.

(Sources: William D. McArdle, Frank I. Katch, Victor L. Katch, *Exercise Physiology: Energy, Nutrition and Human Performance (2nd edition)*, Lea & Febiger, Philadelphia, 1986; and Melvin H. Williams, *Nutrition for Fitness and Sport*, William C. Brown Company Publishers, Dubuque, 1983.)

CONCLUSION

By now I hope that you have a better understanding of the PRIME operating system for YOU 1.0. Together your body and mind act like a computer, only thousands of times more complex. Your mind and body are linked by your nervous system which processes information, relays signals, and initiates actions. Like every other living organism on earth, you operate on certain principles. You must have proper **Posture** which dictates your physical structure. You require **Rest** and downtime to organize and "de-bug." You need food or **Intake** which is your fuel source and input. You must have mental stability within your **Mind** to provide a solid platform to control activity. **Exercise** is essential to become stronger, more resilient, and more physically capable. Without an integration of these components you cannot flourish and reach your maximum potential.

You have been given the ultimate tool to not only survive in this world but also to thrive, a mind and body that is capable of almost anything. In order to ensure your health and well being you need to take care of yourself, just like you would take care of any valuable possession. When YOU 1.0 wear out, you can't go out and get a new body, mind, or soul. There is no extended warranty on you. You have only *one* body, *one* mind, and *one* soul. Don't let life pull the plug before you are ready. With a little effort you will never become outdated or obsolete. You can and will continue to update and get better and better.

TROUBLE SHOOTING GUIDE FOR YOU 1.0

Our own physical body possesses a wisdom which we who inhabit the body lack. We give it orders which make no sense.

Henry Miller

The following is a trouble shooting guide for YOU 1.0. If you should experience any of the problems listed below try the remedies listed or seek the advice of your physician. If you believe that you have an emergency call 911.

Trouble Shooting Guide

Problem	Possible Cause	Try this
Burn	Heat Source	Cool water on the burn. NO BUTTER. Wrap with sterile gauze and seek medical attention.
Cold/Flu	You 1.0 infected by a virus or bacteria	Increase water intake, rest, and fruit consumption. Decrease physical activity and sugar consumption. Wash hands frequently. Gargle with salt water for sore throat. Zinc and Echinacea may be helpful. (Read precautions on all nutritional supplement labels and talk to your physician.)
Constipation	Medications, lack of fiber, decreased fluid intake, inactivity.	Increase water intake, fiber, fruits, and vegetables. Initiate a diet change and an exercise program.

Problem	Possible Cause	Try This
Depression	Stress, hormonal imbalance, environmental factors, medications, nutrient deficiency, biochemical abnormalities, other causes.	Initiate a diet and exercise program, seek professional help. New treatments are very effective.
Diarrhea	Gastric inflammation, food poisoning, gastric hypermotility	Increase water intake. Avoid caffeine, alcohol, and dairy products. Initiate B.R.A.T. diet: Bananas, Rice, Apple Sauce, and Toast. If food poisoning, let run its course. If lasts more than a few days seek medical attention.
Fatigue	Many causes. Allergies, medications, medical conditions, nutrition.	Initiate diet and exercise program. Increase intake of fruits and vegetables, fiber, and water. Decrease fried foods, refined sugars and carbohydrates, alcohol, and caffeine. Increase quality sleep. If condition persists seek medical attention to determine cause.

Problem	Possible Cause	Try This
Fever	Natural immune response to infection	Luke warm bath (not cold). Increase water intake. No aspirin for children. Seek medical attention if over 103 degrees.
Fibromyalgia (Muscle Pain)	Not known. Possible hormonal/chemical imbalance may contribute.	Increase intake of water, dark leafy green vegetables, fish, beans, whole grains, and fruits (except citrus). Increase quality sleep. Decrease intake of soda, red meat, alcohol, caffeine, dairy, MSG, nuts, refined sugars and carbohydrates. Acupuncture, chiropractic, and massage may be helpful.
Headaches	May be caused by stress, tension, tobacco, alcohol, environment, medical condition, hormones, posture, blood sugar levels, allergies, TMJ problems.	Improve posture. Increase water intake. Acupuncture, chiropractic, and massage may be helpful. Improve sleep habits. Try to avoid triggers such as MSG, alcohol, caffeine, sugar, and chocolate.

Problem	Possible Cause	Try This
High blood pressure	Specific cause unknown	Initiate exercise and diet modification. Self monitor blood pressure. Decrease weight, stress levels, alcohol consumption (2 per day). Quit smoking.
Heartburn	Gastric irritation	Eat at least 3 hours before bed time or laying on back. Avoid tight clothing (ie: neck tie, tight shirt/pants). Chew food thoroughly. Decrease intake of spicy, dairy, citrus, high fat foods. Avoid alcohol, tobacco, caffeine.
Insomnia	Medications, physical, medical, psychological problems	Try to sleep on a good quality mattress and pillow. Relax 1 hour before and no exercise within 3 hours of bedtime. Decrease caffeine intake and large meals before bedtime. Decrease stress, avoid naps during the day. Avoid falling to sleep with T.V. on.

Problem	Possible Cause	Try This
Minor Cut/Abrasion	Many causes possible	Keep level of cut above heart and keep pressure directly on cut until bleeding stops. Use soap and clean water to clean wound, do not use hydrogen peroxide. Put clean bandage on wound. Seek medical attention if necessary.
Muscle Stiffness	Overexertion, Medical Cause, Subluxation	Massage and Chiropractic may be helpful. Avoid sudden movements. Increase fruit and vegetable intake. Gentle stretching. R.I.C.E.-Rest, Ice, Compression, Elevation.
Poison Ivy	Direct or Indirect Contact with Poison Ivy	Avoid 3 leafed plants. Avoid itching and wash affected areas with soap and water. Calamine lotion may reduce the irritation. Wash clothes worn outdoors.

Problem	Possible Cause	Try This
Premenstrual Syndrome	Multiple factors, (including males.)	Initiate exercise and diet modification. Increase intake of fruits, vegetables, fiber, whole grains, and protein. Decrease intake of salt, caffeine, alcohol, red meat, and sugar. Reduce stress.
Stress	Environmental, emotional, and psychological factors.	Initiate diet and exercise modification. Increase intake of fruits and vegetables. Decrease intake of alcohol, caffeine, tobacco, dairy, sugar, and high fat content foods. Modify sleeping habits. Find and focus on activities that reduce stress. Keep a daily journal to establish what triggers stress. Consider enrolling in a support group.

Problem	Possible Cause	Try This
Sunburn	Too much ultraviolet light.	Use sunscreen and wear protective clothing when outdoors, even on cloudy days. If sunburned, increase intake of water. Aloe Vera and cool compress may relieve pain.
Weight Management	Many causes from psychological to physical including depression, increased insulin secretion, excessive calorie intake, hypothyroidism.	Take multifaceted approach. Initiate diet and exercise modification. Increase intake of fruits and vegetables, fiber and whole grains. Avoid "fad" diets. Avoid empty calories and snacks. Decrease intake of sugars and refined carbohydrates. Eat slowly and enjoy your food. Join support group and work with your health care provider.

0-595-34323-6

www.ingramcontent.com/pod-product-compliance
Lightning Source LLC
Chambersburg PA
CBHW020237290526
45784CB00003B/1015